9780781782227

THE 5-MINUTE VETERINARY CONSULT
CANINE AND FELINE SPECIALTY
HANDBOOK

Musculoskeletal Disorders

THE 5-MINUTE VETERINARY CONSULT
CANINE AND FELINE SPECIALTY
HANDBOOK

Musculoskeletal Disorders

Consulting Editor

Peter K. Shires, BVSc, MS
Diplomate ACVS
Professor
Department of Small Animal Surgery
Virginia-Maryland Regional
College of Veterinary Medicine, Blacksburg, Virginia

Co-Editor
Larry Patrick Tilley, DVM
Diplomate, American College of Veterinary
Internal Medicine (Internal Medicine)
President, VetMed Consultants
Chief Medical Officer, Dr. Tilley & Associates
Sante Fe, New Mexico

Co-Editor
Francis W. K. Smith, Jr., DVM
Diplomate, American College of Veterinary
Internal Medicine (Internal Medicine & Cardiology)
Vice-President, VetMed Consultants
Lexington, Massachusetts
Clinical Assistant Professor, Department of Medicine
Tufts University, School of Veterinary Medicine
North Grafton, Massachusetts
Executive Editor: David B. Troy

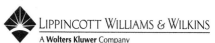

LIPPINCOTT WILLIAMS & WILKINS
A **Wolters Kluwer** Company
Philadelphia • Baltimore • New York • London
Buenos Aires • Hong Kong • Sydney • Tokyo

Managing Editor: Rebecca A. Kerins
Project Editor: Christina Remsberg
Marketing Manager: Marisa O'Brien
Designer: Teresa Mallon
Compositor: Maryland Composition
Printer: RR Donnelley-Crawfordsville

The publisher is not responsible (as a matter of product liability, negligence,
or otherwise) for any injury resulting from any material contained herein.
This publication contains information relating to general principles of medical care that should not be construed as specific instructions for individual
patients. Manufacturers' product information and package inserts should
be reviewed for current information, including contraindications, dosages,
and precautions.

Printed in the United States of America

Library of Congress Cataloging-in-Publication Data

LOC data is available (0-7817-8222-8)

The publishers have made every effort to trace the copyright holders for
borrowed material. If they have inadvertently overlooked any, they will be
pleased to make the necessary arrangements at the first opportunity.

To purchase additional copies of this book, call our customer service
department at (800) 638-3030 or fax orders to (301) 824-7390.
International customers should call (301) 714-2324.

Visit Lippincott Williams & Wilkins on the Internet:
http://www.LWW.com. Lippincott Williams & Wilkins customer service
representatives are available from 8:30 am to 6:00 pm, EST.

05 06 07 08 09
1 2 3 4 5 6 7 8 9 10

Preface

Keeping abreast of advances in the various specialties in veterinary internal medicine is extremely difficult, especially for the busy general practitioner. *The 5-Minute Veterinary Consult Canine and Feline Specialty Handbook: Musculoskeletal* is designed to provide the busy veterinary practitioner and student with a concise, practical review of almost all of the diseases and clinical problems relating to the musculoskeletal system in dogs and cats. Emphasis is placed on diagnosis and treatment of musculoskeletal problems and diseases likely to be seen by veterinarians.

The uniqueness and value of this handbook as a quick reference is the consistency of presentation, the breadth of coverage, and the contribution of a large number of experts. The format of every topic is identical, making it easy to find information.

As the title implies, one objective of this handbook is to make information quickly available. To this end, we have organized topics alphabetically. Most topics can be found without using the index. Illustrations are also included, depicting anatomy and certain diseases and conditions. This handbook and included images brings to the clinic examination room an easy-to-use medical resource that will improve your expertise in diseases and conditions related to the musculoskeletal system in dogs and cats.

This series of specialty handbooks constitutes an important, up-to-date medical reference source for your practice and clinical education. We strive to make it complete yet practical and easy to use. Our dreams are realized if this text helps you to quickly locate and use the "momentarily important" information that is essential to the practice of high-quality veterinary medicine.

Drs. Peter Shires, Larry Tilley, and Frank Smith
c/o Lippincott Williams & Wilkins
Baltimore, Maryland

Acknowledgments

The editors gratefully acknowledge the contributors who, by their expertise, have so unmistakably enhanced the quality of this handbook.

A special thank you goes to all of the staff at Lippincott Williams & Wilkins and everyone in the production and editing departments. The marketing and sales departments also must be acknowledged for generating such an interest in this book. They are all meticulous workers and kind people who have made the final stages of preparing this book both inspiring and fun. An important life goal of ours has been fulfilled: to provide expertise in small animal musculoskeletal medicine and to teach the principles contained in this handbook to veterinarians and students everywhere.

Lippincott Williams & Wilkins would also like to acknowledge the following sources for the images provided in the color insert. Images on pages 1–14 provided courtesy of Anatomical Chart Company. Images on pages 15 and 16 are from *Stedman's Medical Dictionary, 27th Edition With Veterinary Medicine Insert,* Baltimore, MD, Lippincott Williams & Wilkins, 2004.

Contributors

Brian S. Beale, DVM Diplomate, ACVS, Gulf Coast Veterinary Surgery, Houston, Texas

Jamie R. Bellah, DVM Diplomate, ACVS, Adjunct Professor, University of Florida, Staff Surgeon, Affiliated Veterinary Specialists—Orange Park, Orange Park, Florida

Larry G. Carpenter, DVM, MS Diplomate, ACVS, Surgeon, Department of Defense Military Working Dog Center, Veterinary Services, Lackland Air Force Base, San Antonio, Texas

Georgina Child, BVSc Diplomate, ACVIM (Neurology), Veterinary Specialist (Neurology), Veterinary Specialist Centre, North Ryde, New South Wales, Australia

Erick L. Egger, DVM Diplomate ACVS, Affiliate Faculty, Veterinary Orthopedic Consultant, Clinical Sciences, Colorado State University, Fort Collins, Colorado

Scott P. Hammel, DVM Resident in Small Animal Surgery, College of Veterinary Medicine, University of Minnesota, St. Paul, Minnesota

Kenneth A. Johnson MVSc, PhD, FACVSc. Diplomate, ACVS, Diplomate, ECVS, Professor of Orthopaedics, Department of Veterinary Clinical Science, The Ohio State University, Columbus, Ohio

Spencer A. Johnston, VMD Diplomate, ACVS Professor, Small Animal Surgery, Department of Small Animal Clinical Sciences, Virginia-Maryland Regional College of Veterinary Medicine, Blacksburg, Virginia

CONTRIBUTORS

Otto I. Lanz, DVM   Diplomate ACVS, Assistant Professor, Department of Small Animal Clinical Sciences, Virginia-Maryland Regional College of Veterinary Medicine, Blacksburg, Virginia

Ron McLaughlin, DVM, DVSc   Diplomate, ACVS Associate Professor and Chief, Small Animal Surgery, Department of Clinical Sciences, College of Veterinary Medicine, Mississippi State University,Mississippi State, Mississippi

Gary D. Osweiler, DVM, PhD   Diplomate, ABVT Professor / Director, Veterinary Diagnostic & Production Animal Medicine / Veterinary Diagnostic Laboratory, Iowa State University, Ames, Iowa

Peter D. Schwarz, DVM   Diplomate, ACVS, Veterinary Surgical Specialists of New Mexico, Albuquerque, New Mexico

G. Diane Shelton, DVM, PhD   Diplomate, ACVIM (Internal Medicine), Adjunct Professor, Department of Pathology, University of California, San Diego, LaJolla, California

Peter K. Shires, BVSc, MS   Diplomate, ACVS, Professor, Department of Small Animal Surgery, Virginia-Maryland Regional College of Veterinary Medicine, Blacksburg, Virginia

Mark M. Smith, VMD   Diplomate, ACVS, AVDC Professor and Chief of Small Animal Surgery, Department of Small Animal Clinical Sciences, Virginia-Maryland Regional College of Veterinary Medicine, Blacksburg, Virginia

William B. Thomas, DVM, MS   Diplomate, ACVIM (Neurology), Associate Professor, Department of Small

Animal Clinical Sciences, University of Tennessee, Knoxville, Tennessee

Don R. Waldron, DVM   Diplomate, ACVS, ABVp Professor of Surgery, Department of Small Animal Clinical Sciences, Virginia-Maryland Regional College of Veterinary Medicine, Blacksburg, Virginia

Jennifer Warnock   Gulf Coast Veterinary Surgery, Houston, Texas

Ronald B. Wilson, DVM   Diplomate, ACVP, Laboratory Director, C.E. Cord Animal Disease, Diagnostic Laboratory, Tennessee Department of Agriculture, Nashville, Tennessee

Deanna Worley, DVM   Gulf Coast Veterinary Surgery, Houston, Texas

Contents

CONTENTS

Antebrachial Growth Deformities

 BASICS

DEFINITION
Abnormally shaped forelimbs and/or malalignments of the elbow or antebrachial carpal joints that result from abnormal development of the radius or ulna in the growing animal

PATHOPHYSIOLOGY
- Antebrachium—predisposed to deformities resulting from continual growth of one bone after premature growth cessation or decreased growth rate of the paired bone
- Decreased rate of elongation in one bone behaves as a retarding strap; the growing paired bone must twist and bow away from the short bone or overgrow at the elbow or carpus; causes joint malalignment
- Normal growth—bones elongate through the process of endochondral ossification, which occurs in the physis; physis closure occurs when the germinal cell layer stops producing new cartilage and the existing cartilage hypertrophies, ossifies, and is remodeled into bone.
- Hereditary—premature closure of distal ulnar physis reported as recessive trait in Skye terriers; may be a component of common elbow joint malalignment in many chondrodysplastic breeds (basset hounds and lhasa apsos)
- Osteochondrosis or dietary oversupplementation—possibly associated with retardation of endochondral ossification (retained cartilaginous cores) in giant-breed dogs
- Trauma—most common cause; if chondroproliferative layer of the physis is crushed (Salter V fracture), new cartilage production and bone elongation are stopped.

SYSTEMS AFFECTED
Musculoskeletal

1

ANTEBRACHIAL GROWTH DEFORMITIES

GENETICS
- Skye terriers—reported as a recessive inheritable trait
- Chondrodysplastic breeds (dogs)—predisposed to elbow malalignment

INCIDENCE/PREVALENCE
- Traumatic—may occur after forelimb injuries in up to 10% of actively growing animals; uncommon in cats
- Elbow malalignment syndrome (chondrodysplastic dog breeds)—fairly common and can be bilateral
- Nutritionally induced—incidence decreasing as nutritional standards are improved
- Congenital agenesis of the radius (cats)—occasionally seen; results in severely bowed antebrachium and carpal subluxation

GEOGRAPHIC DISTRIBUTION
N/A

SIGNALMENT

Species
Dogs and cats

Breed Predilections
- Skye terriers—recessive inheritable form
- Chondrodysplastic and toy breeds (especially basset hounds, dachshunds, lhasa apsos, Pekingese)—may be predisposed to elbow malalignments
- Giant breeds (e.g., great Danes, wolfhounds)—may be induced by rapid growth owing to excessive or unbalanced nutrition

Mean Age and Range
- Traumatic—anytime during the active growth phase
- Elbow malarticulations—during growth; may not be recognized until secondary arthritic changes become severe, occasionally at several years of age

Predominant Sex
N/A

SIGNS

General Comments

- Longer-limbed dogs—angular deformities generally more common
- Shorter-limbed dogs—tend to develop more severe joint malalignments
- Age at the time of premature closure—affects relative degree of deformity and joint malarticulation; perhaps because of the variation in stiffness of bone with age and the duration of altered growth until maturity

Historical Findings

- Traumatic—progressive limb angulation or lameness 3–4 weeks after injury; owner may not be aware of causative event.
- Developmental elbow malalignments—insidious onset of lameness in one or both forelimbs; most apparent after exercise

Physical Examination Findings

Premature Distal Ulnar Closure

- Three deformities of the distal radius—lateral deviation (valgus), cranial bowing (curvus), and external rotation (supination)
- Relative shortening of limb length compared to the contralateral normally growing limb
- Caudolateral subluxation of the radial carpal joint and malarticulation of the elbow joint—may occur; causes lameness and painful joint restriction

Premature Radial Physeal Closure

- Affected limb—significantly shorter than the normal contralateral
- Severity of lameness—depends on degree of joint malarticulation
- Complete symmetrical closure of distal physis—may note straight limb with a widened radial carpal joint space; may note caudal bow to radius and ulna
- Asymmetrical closure of medial distal physis—varus angular deformity; occasionally inward rotation

ANTEBRACHIAL GROWTH DEFORMITIES

- Closure of lateral distal physis—valgus angular deformity; external rotation
- Closure of proximal radial physis with continued ulnar growth—malarticulation of the elbow joint; widened radial to humeral space and humeral to anconeal space

CAUSES
- Trauma
- Developmental basis
- Nutritional basis

RISK FACTORS
- Forelimb trauma
- Excessive dietary supplementation

 DIAGNOSIS

DIFFERENTIAL DIAGNOSIS
- Elbow dysplasia
- Fragmented medial coronoid process
- Un-united anconeal process
- Panosteitis
- Flexor tendon contracture
- Hypertrophic osteodystrophy

CBC/BIOCHEMISTRY/URINALYSIS
N/A

OTHER LABORATORY TESTS
N/A

IMAGING
- Damage to growth potential of the physis—cannot be seen at the time of trauma; usually 2–4 weeks before radiographically apparent
- Standard craniocaudal and mediolateral radiographic views—include entire elbow joint; proximally extend to midmetacarpal level distally; take same series for comparison to normal contralateral limb.
- Degree of angular deformities and relative shortening—determined by comparing relative lengths of radius and

ulna within the deformed pair to the normal contralateral pair
- Elbow and carpal joints—evaluate for malalignment (treated surgically) and arthritis (e.g., osteophytes; influences prognosis)
- Elbow joint—evaluate for associated un-united anconeal process and fragmented medial coronoid process

DIAGNOSTIC PROCEDURES
N/A

PATHOLOGIC FINDINGS
Cartilage of prematurely closed physis replaced with bone

 TREATMENT

APPROPRIATE HEALTH CARE
- Genetic predisposition—cannot be treated
- Traumatic physeal damage—not seen at time of injury; revealed 2–4 weeks later
- Surgical treatment is recommended as soon as possible following diagnosis.

NURSING CARE
N/A

ACTIVITY
Exercise restriction—reduces joint malalignment damage; slows arthritic progression

DIET
- Decrease nutritional supplementation in giant breed dogs—slows rapid growth; may reduce incidence
- Avoid excess weight—helps control arthritic pain resulting from joint malalignment and overuse

CLIENT EDUCATION
- Discuss heritability in Skye terriers and chondrodysplastic breeds.
- Explain that damage to physeal growth potential is not apparent at time of forelimb trauma and that the diagnosis is often made at 2–4-weeks following an injury.

ANTEBRACHIAL GROWTH DEFORMITIES

- Discuss the importance of joint malalignment and result-ant arthritis as primary causes of lameness.
- Emphasize that early surgical treatment leads to a better prognosis.

SURGICAL CONSIDERATIONS

- Premature distal ulnar physeal closure in a patient < 5–6 months of age (significant amount of radial growth potential remaining)—treated with a segmental ulnar ostectomy, valgus deformities ≤ 25°—often sponta-neously correct and may not require additional surgery, young patients and those with more severe deformities—often require a second definitive correction after maturity
- Radial or ulnar physeal closure in a mature patient (limit-ed or no growth potential) requires deformity correction, joint realignment, or both.
- Deformity correction—may be accomplished with a vari-ety of osteotomy techniques; may be stabilized with sev-eral different fixation devices; must correct both rotation-al and angular deformities; performed at the point of greatest curvature
- Joint malalignment (particularly elbow)—must correct to minimize arthritic development (primary cause of lame-ness); obtain optimal joint alignment via dynamic proxi-mal ulnar osteotomy (uses triceps muscle traction and joint pressure).
- Significant limb length discrepancies—distraction osteo-genesis; osteotomy of the shortened bone is progres-sively distracted at the rate of 1 mm/day with an external fixator system to create new bone length.

 MEDICATIONS

DRUG(S) OF CHOICE
Anti-inflammatory drugs—symptomatic treatment of arthritis

CONTRAINDICATIONS
Corticosteroids—do not use owing to potential systemic side effects and cartilage damage seen with long-term use.

PRECAUTIONS
Warn client of possible gastrointestinal upset associated with chronic anti-inflammatory therapy.

POSSIBLE INTERACTIONS
N/A

ALTERNATIVE DRUG(S)
Neutraceuticals (e.g., glycosamines)—may help minimize cartilage damage and arthritis development; may be anti-inflammatory and analgesic

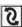 **FOLLOW-UP**

PATIENT MONITORING
- Postoperative—depends on surgical treatment
- Periodic checkups—evaluate arthritic status and anti-inflammatory therapy

PREVENTION/AVOIDANCE
Avoid dietary oversupplementation in rapidly growing giant-breed dogs.

POSSIBLE COMPLICATIONS
Routinely seen with various osteotomy fixation techniques (e.g., infection, nonunion of osteotomy, fixator pin tract inflammation)

EXPECTED COURSE AND PROGNOSIS
- Generally, best results seen with early diagnosis and surgical treatment—minimizes arthritis
- Premature ulnar closure—tends to be easier to manage; yields better results
- Limb lengthening by distraction osteogenesis—requires extensive postoperative management by the veterinarian and owner; high rate of complications

 MISCELLANEOUS

ASSOCIATED CONDITIONS
Osteochondrosis

ANTEBRACHIAL GROWTH DEFORMITIES

AGE-RELATED FACTORS
The younger the age at the time of traumatically induced physeal closure, the more severe the deformity and malarticulation.

ZOONOTIC POTENTIAL
N/A

PREGNANCY
N/A

SYNONYMS
Radius curvus

Suggested Reading

Forrell EB, Schwarz PD. Use of external skeletal fixation for treatment of angular deformity secondary to premature distal ulnar physeal closure. J Am Anim Hosp Assoc 1993;29:460–465.

Gilson SD, Piermattei DL, Schwarz PD. Treatment of humeroulnar subluxation with a dynamic proximal ulnar osteotomy: a review of 13 cases. Vet Surg 1989;18:114–122.

Henney LH, Gambardella PC. Premature closure of the ulnar physis in the dog: a retrospective clinical study. J Am Anim Hosp Assoc 1989;25:573–581.

Johnson AL. Correction of radial and ulnar growth deformities resulting from premature physeal closure. In: Bojrab MJ, ed. Current techniques in small animal surgery. 3rd ed. Philadelphia: Lea & Febiger, 1990:793–801.

Johnson KA. Retardation of endochondral ossification at the distal ulnar growth plate in dogs. Austral Vet J 1981;57:474–478.

Lau RE. Inherited premature closure of the distal ulnar physis. J Am Anim Hosp Assoc 1978;14:690–697.

Yanoff SR, Hulse DA, Palmer RH, Herron MR. Distraction osteogenesis using modified external fixation devices in five dogs. Vet Surg 1992;21:480–486.

Author: Erick L. Egger
Consulting Editor: Peter K. Shires

Arthritis (Degenerative Joint Disease)

 BASICS

DEFINITION
Degenerative joint disease (DJD) is the progressive and permanent deterioration of the articular cartilage of diarthrodial (synovial) joints due to primary (idiopathic) and secondary causes.

PATHOPHYSIOLOGY
- DJD is classified as a noninflammatory joint disease because the initial disease process is not driven by inflammatory mediators; however, inflammation is strongly correlated with the progression of DJD.
- Metalloproteinases, serine proteases, and cysteine protease enzymes are released from damaged chondrocytes, causing collagen degradation and loss of collagen crosslinking in cartilage.
- Collagen synthesis is altered by production of an abnormal type XI collagen and ratio of type II collagen, resulting in decreased collagen/proteoglycan interaction and weakened collagen structure.
- Cartilage matrix is further weakened by increased breakdown of proteoglycans and production of structurally abnormal proteoglycans.
- Nitric oxide (NO) is also released, which mediates cartilage breakdown and supports chronic inflammation. Chondrocyte apoptosis is mediated by cyclooxygenase-2 enzymes and inducible NO synthase.
- Inflammation causes decreased elasticity and viscosity of the synovial fluid, resulting in increased contact friction and pain.
- Subchondral bone becomes sclerotic, reducing bone elasticity and worsening mechanical impact on articular cartilage.

ARTHRITIS (DEGENERATIVE JOINT DISEASE)

- Pain of DJD results from stimulation of Aδ and C fibers in the tendons, ligament, subchondral bone, and joint capsule. Pain is chemically mediated by prostaglandins, leukotrienes, substance P, bradykinin, and cytokines.
- The result of these processes is progressive cartilage degradation ranging from fibrillation to deep fissuring of cartilage. Full thickness cartilage loss can eventually occur.

SYSTEMS AFFECTED
Musculoskeletal—diarthrodial joints

GENETICS
- Primary DJD has been associated with a colony of beagles.
- Dogs—causes of secondary DJD are likely inheritable, including elbow dysplasia in rottweilers, osteochondrosis dissecans in Bernese mountain dogs, hip dysplasia in large-breed (e.g., German shepherds, Labradors) and small-breed dogs (e.g., cocker spaniels, Shetland sheepdogs), patellar luxation in small and miniature-breed dogs, congenital shoulder luxation and elbow luxation in small-breed dogs.
- Cats—causes of secondary DJD are likely inheritable, such as patellar luxation in the Devon rex, hip dysplasia in Siamese and other breeds, and arthropathy in Scottish folds.

INCIDENCE/PREVALENCE
- Dogs—likely the most common skeletal disease; estimated that 20% of dogs older than 1 year have some degree of DJD. Actual incidence unknown.
- Cats—one study reported that of 100 cats over 12 years of age presenting for nonmusculoskeletal disease, 90% had evidence of osteoarthritis on radiographs. Actual incidence unknown.
- Secondary DJD is much more common than primary DJD.

SIGNALMENT

Species
Dogs and cats

Breed Predilections
None

ARTHRITIS (DEGENERATIVE JOINT DISEASE)

Mean Age and Range
- Primary—usually older animals
- Hereditary and congenital disorders, such as osteochondrosis, seen in immature animals; hip dysplasia can present bimodally at young and old age
- Trauma induced—any age

Predominant Sex
None

SIGNS

Historical Findings

Dogs
- Decrease in activity level or willingness to perform certain tasks; intermittent lameness or stiff gait that slowly becomes more severe and frequent
- May have a history of previous joint trauma, osteochondral disease, or developmental disorder
- May be exacerbated by exercise, long periods of recumbency, and cold weather

Cats
- Overt lameness may not be noted.
- May have difficulty grooming, jumping onto furniture, or getting in and out of the litter box; overall increase in irritability

Physical Examination Findings
- Stiffness of gait
- Altered gait (e.g., bunny hopping in hip dysplasia)
- Lameness
- Decreased range of motion
- Crepitus
- Joint swelling (effusion and thickening of the joint capsule)
- Joint pain
- Joint instability (ligament tears, subluxation), depending on duration of disease
- Gross joint deformity

CAUSES
- Articular cartilage has limited ability to repair and regenerate in response to low-grade wear and tear, trauma,

11

ARTHRITIS (DEGENERATIVE JOINT DISEASE)

instability, abnormal weight bearing, abnormalities in cartilage structure, or joint incongruity.

- Primary—thought to be the result of long-term use combined with aging; no known predisposing cause
- Secondary—results from an initiating cause: abnormal wear on normal cartilage (e.g., joint instability, joint incongruity, trauma to cartilage or supporting soft tissues) or normal wear on abnormal cartilage (e.g., osteochondral defects)

RISK FACTORS
- Working, athletic, and obese dogs place more stress on their joints.
- Dogs with Cushing's disease, diabetes mellitus, or hypothyroidism may be more prone owing to decreased anabolic capability and increased catabolic processes.

 DIAGNOSIS

DIFFERENTIAL DIAGNOSIS
- Neoplastic (synovial cell sarcoma; rarely, chondrosarcoma; osteosarcoma)
- Infectious arthritis (caused by bacteria; spirochetes; L-forms in cats; *Mycoplasma*; *Rickettsia*; *Ehrlichia*; viruses, such as feline calicivirus; fungi, and protozoa)
- Immune mediated (erosive vs. nonerosive)

CBC/BIOCHEMISTRY/URINALYSIS
N/A

OTHER LABORATORY TESTS
- Coombs' test, ANA, and rheumatoid factor may help to rule out immune-mediated arthritis.
- Serum titers for *Borrelia*, *Ehrlichia*, and *Rickettsia* to evaluate for infectious arthritis

IMAGING
- Radiographic changes—include joint capsular distention, osteophytosis, enthesiophytosis, soft tissue thickening, and narrowed joint spaces; in severely affected patients:

subchondral sclerosis, subchondral bone cysts, attrition of subchondral bone, mineralization of joint soft tissues, and intra-articular calcified bodies (joint mice). Radiographic severity often does not correlate with clinical severity.

- Stress radiography may identify underlying instability and accentuate joint incongruity; e.g., distraction index (passive hip laxity) of the coxofemoral joint is predictive of risk of hip DJD.
- Computed tomography can be particularly useful in determining joint incongruence, e.g., elbow dysplasia.
- Ultrasonography can be used to determine ligamentous and tendinous injury (hypoechoic appearance and disruption of normal fibrillar orientation) and has been reported to be useful in identifying soft tissue changes in stifles with cranial cruciate ligament injury.
- Three-phase nuclear scintigraphy of bone can assist in localizing subtle DJD via nucleotide uptake at areas of increased perfusion and bone turnover.

DIAGNOSTIC PROCEDURES
- Arthrocentesis and synovial fluid analysis support the diagnosis—cell counts are normal or slightly increased (< 2000–5000 cells/mL) and predominantly mononuclear (macrophages); synovial lining cells or cartilage fragments occasionally observed
- Large numbers of neutrophils likely the result of underlying immune-mediated or infectious arthritis
- Bacterial culture and sensitivity of synovial fluid—negative
- Biopsy of synovial tissue helps rule out neoplasia or other arthritides, such as lymphocytic plasmacytic synovitis.
- Force plating allows quantitative determination and analysis of weight bearing; vertical peak force and impulse are decreased in joints affected by osteoarthritis.

PATHOLOGIC FINDINGS
- Fibrillation or erosion of articular cartilage
- Eburnation and sclerosis of subchondral bone
- Thickening and fibrosis of the joint capsule

ARTHRITIS (DEGENERATIVE JOINT DISEASE)

- Synovial fluid can be grossly normal to thin and watery, usually increased volume
- Synovial villous hypertrophy and hyperplasia
- Osteophytes and enthesiophytes at joint capsule attachments and adjacent to the joint
- Neovascularization or pannus in severe cases over joint surfaces

 TREATMENT

APPROPRIATE HEALTH CARE
- Medical—usually tried initially
- Surgical options—if inadequate response to medical management

NURSING CARE
- Physical therapy—very beneficial in enhancing good limb function and general well-being
- Passive range of motion exercises
- Massage
- Combination cold and heat therapy
- Swimming—increases range of motion of all joints; aerobic exercise with minimal weight bearing
- Controlled leash walks up hills or on soft surfaces, such as sand

ACTIVITY
Limited to a level that minimizes aggravation of clinical signs

DIET
- Limited food consumption decreases development of clinical and radiographic evidence of DJD.
- Weight reduction for obese patients—decreases stress placed on arthritic joints
- Reduced caloric intake—recommended because of decreased activity as a result of disease and aging
- Avoid nutrient excess and rapid growth in dogs that may be predisposed to underlying developmental diseases (e.g., hip dysplasia and osteochondrosis).

- n-6 and n-3 polyunsaturated fatty acids may decrease the production of certain prostaglandins and modulate inflammation.

CLIENT EDUCATION
- Inform client that medical therapy is palliative and the condition is likely to progress.
- Discuss treatment options, activity level, and diet.

SURGICAL CONSIDERATIONS
- Arthrotomy—used to treat underlying causes (e.g., fragmented coronoid process, ununited anconeal process, osteochondral diseases)
- Arthroscopy—allows actual visualization of articular cartilage; used to diagnose and treat underlying causes; has been described for hip, stifle, hock, shoulder, elbow, and carpus; has added benefit of flushing the joint
- Reconstructive procedures—used to eliminate joint instability and correct anatomic deficiencies (e.g., tibial plateau leveling osteotomy for cranial cruciate ligament–deficient stifles)
- Corrective procedures—used to alter abnormal weight-bearing forces on joints with incongruity (e.g., corrective ulnar osteotomy in dogs with elbow incongruity)

Arthroplasty Procedures
- Commonly performed for hip
- THR—may give excellent results; recommended for dogs that can accommodate the implants
- Femoral head ostectomy—for smaller dogs and cats; selected patients that cannot afford THR
- Total elbow replacement still experimental and offered in select cases

Arthrodesis
- Selected chronic cases and for joint instability
- Complete or partial—based on location of condition or instability
- Carpus—generally yields excellent results
- Shoulder, elbow, stifle, hock—less predictable results

MEDICATIONS

DRUG(S) OF CHOICE

NSAIDs
- Work by inhibiting prostaglandin synthesis by the COX enzyme
- Deracoxib (3–4 mg/kg PO q24h for 7 days for postoperative pain) (1–2 mg/kg PO q24h for long term treatment over 7 days)—new COX-2 inhibitor (coxib) drug that is selective only for the inducible COX-2 enzyme that causes pain and inflammation; spares the constitutive COX-1 enzyme responsible for gastrointestinal health and kidney function
- Carprofen (2.2 mg/kg PO q12h) and etodolac (10–15 mg/kg PO q24h)—more selective for COX-2 and therefore less irritating to the gastrointestinal system; carprofen has also been shown to reduce progression of morphologic changes in cartilage and subchondral bone in canine arthritic joints.
- Buffered aspirin (25 mg/kg PO q12h)
- Meclofenamic acid—0.5 mg/kg PO q12h may also be given
- Cats—limited to aspirin (10 mg/kg PO every 3 days)

Chondroprotective Agents
- Inhibits various destructive enzymes and prostaglandins
- Chondrostimulation—associated with increased production of proteoglycan, hyaluronate, and collagen
- GAGPs (Adequan)—recent clinical study of dogs with hip dysplasia found the greatest improvement in orthopedic scores at 4.4 mg/kg IM every 3–5 days for eight injections

CONTRAINDICATIONS
- NSAIDs must not be given with steroids or to dogs in which steroid therapy is being considered.
- Acetaminophen must not be given to cats.
- NSAIDs must not be given to dogs with renal insufficieny or renal failure, dehydration, hypotension, shock, trauma, hemangiosarcoma, disorders of coagulation, or

gastrointestinal disorders (especially if there is evidence of gastrointestinal ulceration), or to dogs that may undergo surgery for intervertebral disk disease (increased bleeding at the spinal cord).
- NSAIDs and GAGPs—simultaneous use not recommended; potential additive inhibition of hemostasis

PRECAUTIONS
- NSAIDs—decrease platelet function; may cause gastric ulceration; may decrease blood flow to the kidneys; in cases of severe pulmonary disease, may also inhibit bronchiolar muscle relaxation; COX-2 selective drugs may interfere with liver and placental function
- Naproxen, piroxicam, flunixin meglumine, and ibuprofen—their use is discouraged because of ulcerogenic potential

POSSIBLE INTERACTIONS
None known

ALTERNATIVE DRUG(S)
Nutraceuticals and free-radical scavengers

Corticosteroids
- Glucocorticoids—inhibit inflammatory mediators and cytokines; however, chronic use delays healing and initiates damage to articular cartilage; potential systemic side effects documented; goal is low-dose (dogs, 0.5–2.0 mg/kg; cats, 2.0–4.0 mg/kg), alternate-day therapy
- Prednisone—initial dose 1–2 mg/kg PO q24h for dogs and 4 mg/kg PO q24h for cats
- Triamcinolone hexacetonide—intra-articular injection of 5 mg in dogs showed a protective and therapeutic effect in one model

 FOLLOW-UP

PATIENT MONITORING
Clinical deterioration—indicates need to change drug selection or dosage; may indicate need for surgical intervention

ARTHRITIS (DEGENERATIVE JOINT DISEASE)

PREVENTION/AVOIDANCE

Early identification of predisposing causes and prompt treatment to help reduce progression of secondary conditions, e.g., surgical removal of osteochondral lesions

EXPECTED COURSE AND PROGNOSIS

- Slow progression of disease likely
- Some form of medical or surgical treatment usually allows a good quality of life.

 MISCELLANEOUS

SYNONYMS

- Osteoarthritis
- Degenerative joint disease
- Osteoarthrosis
- Degenerative arthritis

ABBREVIATIONS

- ANA = antinuclear antibody
- COX = cyclooxygenase
- DJD = degenerative joint disease
- GAGPs = glycosaminoglycan polysulfate esters
- NO = nitric oxide
- NSAID = nonsteroidal antiinflammatory drug
- THR = total hip replacement

Suggested Readings

Pederson NC. Joint diseases of dogs and cats. In: Ettinger SJ, ed. Textbook of veterinary internal medicine. 5th ed. Philadelphia: Saunders, 2000:1862–1886.

Authors: Brian S. Beale & Jennifer J. Warnock
Section Editor: Peter K. Shires

Arthritis, Septic

 BASICS

DEFINITION
Pathogenic microorganisms within the closed space of one or more synovial joints

PATHOPHYSIOLOGY
- Usually caused by contamination associated with traumatic injury (e.g., a direct penetrating injury such as bite or gunshot wounds), a sequela to surgery, hematogenous spread of microorganisms from a distant septic focus, or the extension of primary osteomyelitis
- Primary sources of hematogenous infection—urogenital, respiratory, integumentary (including ears and anal sacs), respiratory, cardiac, and gastrointestinal systems

SYSTEMS AFFECTED
Musculoskeletal system—usually affects one joint

GENETICS
N/A

INCIDENCE/PREVALENCE
Relatively uncommon cause of monoarticular arthritis in dogs and cats

GEOGRAPHIC DISTRIBUTION
May be an increased incidence in Lyme disease–endemic areas

SIGNALMENT

Species
- Most common in dogs
- Rare in cats

Breed Predilections
Medium to large breeds—most commonly German shepherds, Dobermans, and Labrador retrievers

ARTHRITIS, SEPTIC

Mean Age and Range
Any age; usually between 4 and 7 years

Predominant Sex
Male

SIGNS

General Comments
Always consider the diagnosis in patients with monoarticular lameness associated with soft tissue swelling, heat, and pain.

Historical Findings
- Lameness—acute onset most commonly, but can present as a chronic lameness
- Lethargy
- Anorexia
- May report previous trauma—dog bite, penetrating injury

Physical Examination Findings
- Monoarticular lameness, rarely pauciarticular
- Joint pain and swelling—commonly carpus, stifle, hock, shoulder, or cubital joint
- Localized joint heat
- Decreased range of motion
- Fever

CAUSES
- Aerobic bacterial organisms—most common: staphylococci, streptococci, coliforms, and *Pasteurella*
- Anaerobic organisms—most common: *Propionibacterium, Peptostreptococcus, Fusobacterium,* and *Bacteroides*
- Spirochete—*Borrelia burgdorferi*
- Mycoplasma
- Fungal agents—*Blastomyces,* cryptococcus, and *Coccidiodes*
- *Ehrlichia*
- Leishmania

RISK FACTORS
- Predisposing factors for hematogenous infection— diabetes mellitus; Addison disease; immunosuppression

- Penetrating trauma to the joint
- Existing osteoarthritis or other joint damage
- Intra-articular injection, particularly if steroid injected

 DIAGNOSIS

DIFFERENTIAL DIAGNOSIS
- Osteoarthritis
- Trauma
- Immune-mediated arthropathy
- Postvaccinal transient polyarthritis
- Greyhound polyarthritis
- Crystal-induced joint disease
- Synovial cell sarcoma

CBC/BIOCHEMISTRY/URINALYSIS
- Hemogram—inflammatory left shift
- Other results normal

OTHER LABORATORY TESTS
Serologic testing for specific pathogens

IMAGING

Radiography
- Early disease—may reveal thickened and dense periarticular tissues; may see evidence of synovial effusion. Often difficult to diagnose early disease radiographically
- Late disease—reveals bone destruction, osteolysis, irregular joint space, discrete erosions, and periarticular osteophytosis

DIAGNOSTIC PROCEDURES

Synovial Fluid Analysis
- Increased volume
- Turbid fluid
- Decreased mucin clot reaction
- Elevated WBC count—$> 80\%$ neutrophils with $> 40,000/mm^3$ (normal joint fluid $< 10\%$ neutrophils and $< 3,000/mm^3$).
- Bacteria in the synovial fluid or within neutrophils—show toxic changes (chromatolysis, nuclear swelling, loss of

segmentation). However, toxic neutrophils are not necessary for diagnosis.

Synovial Fluid Culture

- Culture definitive for diagnosis
- Must be collected aseptically; requires heavy sedation or general anesthesia
- Place fluid sample in aerobic and anaerobic Culturettes and in blood culture medium
- Use 1:9 dilution of synovial fluid to blood culture media.
- Culturette samples—cultured immediately upon arrival to the laboratory
- Blood culture medium—re-culturing after 24 hr of incubation increases accuracy by 50% and is the preferred method.

Other

- Synovial biopsy—to rule out immune-mediated joint disease; no more effective than culturing incubated blood culture medium
- Blood and urine cultures if hematogenous source is suspected

PATHOLOGIC FINDINGS

- Synovium—thickened; discolored; often very proliferative
- Histology—evidence of hyperplastic synoviocytes
- Increased numbers of neutrophils, macrophages, and fibrinous debris
- Cartilage—loss of proteoglycan, destruction of articular surface, pannus formation

 TREATMENT

APPROPRIATE HEALTH CARE

- Inpatient—initial stabilization; initiate systemic antibiotic therapy as soon as fluid is obtained for bacterial culture; initiate joint drainage/lavage as soon as possible to minimize intra-articular injury.
- Identify source if hematogenous spread is suspected.
- Outpatient—long-term management

NURSING CARE
Alternating heat and cold packing—beneficial in promoting increased blood flow and decreased swelling

ACTIVITY
Restricted until resolution of symptoms

DIET
N/A

CLIENT EDUCATION
- Discuss probable cause.
- Warn client about the need for long-term antibiotics and the likelihood of residual degenerative joint disease.

SURGICAL CONSIDERATIONS
- Acute disease with minimal radiogaphic changes—joint drainage and lavage via needle arthrocentesis, arthroscopic lavage, or arthrotomy. An irrigation catheter (ingress/egress) can be placed in larger joints
- Chronic disease—requires open arthrotomy with débridement of the synovium and copious lavage; place an irrigation catheter (ingress/egress) to lavage the joint postoperatively.
- Lavage—use warmed physiologic saline or lactated Ringer's solution (2–4 ml/kg q8h) until effluent is clear. Do not add povidone/iodine or chlorhexidine to lavage fluid.
- Effluent fluid—cytologically monitored daily for existence and character of bacteria and neutrophils
- Removal of catheters—when effluent fluid has no bacteria and the neutrophils are cytologically healthy

 MEDICATIONS

DRUG(S) OF CHOICE
- Pending culture susceptibility data—bactericidal antibiotics, such as first-generation cephalosporin or ampicillin–clavulanic acid, preferred
- Choice of antimicrobial drugs—primarily depends on in vitro determination of susceptibility of microorganisms; toxicity, frequency, route of administration, and expense

also considered; most penetrate the synovium well; need to be given for a minimum of 4–8 weeks
- NSAIDs—may help decrease pain and inflammation

CONTRAINDICATIONS
Avoid quinolones in pediatric patients; they induce cartilage lesions experimentally.

PRECAUTIONS
Failure to respond to conventional antibiotic therapy—may indicate anaerobic disease or other unusual cause (fungal, spirochete)

POSSIBLE INTERACTIONS
N/A

ALTERNATIVE DRUG(S)
N/A

 FOLLOW-UP

PATIENT MONITORING
- Drainage and irrigation catheters—may be pulled after 4–6 days or after reassessment of synovial fluid cytology
- Duration of antibiotic therapy—2 weeks following resolution of clinical signs. Total treatment may be 4–8 weeks or longer; depends on clinical signs and pathogenic organism
- Persistent synovial inflammation without viable bacterial organisms (dogs)—may be caused by antigenic bacterial fragments or antigen antibody deposition
- Systemic corticosteroid therapy and aggressive physical therapy—may be needed to maximize normal joint dynamics

PREVENTION/AVOIDANCE
If clinical signs recur, early (within 24–48 hr) treatment provides the greatest benefit.

POSSIBLE COMPLICATIONS
- Chronic disease—severe degenerative joint disease
- Recurrence of infection
- Limited joint range of motion

- Generalized sepsis
- Osteomyelitis

EXPECTED COURSE AND PROGNOSIS
- Acutely diagnosed disease (within 24–48 hr) responds well to antibiotic therapy
- Delayed diagnosis or resistant or highly virulent organisms—guarded to poor prognosis

 MISCELLANEOUS

ASSOCIATED CONDITIONS
N/A

AGE-RELATED FACTORS
N/A

ZOONOTIC POTENTIAL
N/A

PREGNANCY
N/A

SYNONYMS
- Infectious arthritis
- Joint ill

SEE ALSO
- Osteomyelitis
- Polyarthritis, Erosive Immune-Mediated
- Polyarthritis, Nonerosive Immune-Mediated

ABBREVIATION
- NSAIDS = nonsteroidal antiinflammatory drugs

Suggested Reading
Bennett D, Taylor DJ. Bacterial infective arthritis in the dog. J Small Anim Pract 1988;29:207–230.

Ellison RS. The cytologic examination of synovial fluid. Semin Vet Med Surg Small Anim 1988;3:133–139.

Hodgin EC, Michaelson F, Howerth EW. Anaerobic bacterial infections causing osteomyelitis/arthritis in a dog. J Am Vet Med Assoc 1992;201:886–888.

ARTHRITIS, SEPTIC

Machevsky AM, Read RA. Bacterial septic arthritis in 19 dogs. Aust Vet J 1999; 77:233–237.

Montgomery RD, Long IR, Milton JL. Comparison of aerobic Culturette, synovial membrane biopsy, and blood culture medium in detection of canine bacterial arthritis. Vet Surg 1989;18:300–303.

Nord KD, Dore DD, Deeney VF, et al. Evaluation of treatment modalities for septic arthritis with histologic grading and analysis of levels of uronic acid, neutral protease, and interleukin-1. J Bone Jt Surg 1995; 77:258–265.

Acknowledgment

The author/editors acknowledge the prior contributions of Dr. Robert A. Taylor, who authored this topic in the previous edition.

Author: Spencer A. Johnston
Consulting Editor: Peter K. Shires

Atlantoaxial Instability

 BASICS

OVERVIEW
- Results from malformation or disruption of the articulation between the first two cervical vertebrae (atlas and axis); causes spinal cord compression
- Usually associated with a congenital anomaly of the dens (aplasia, hypoplasia, or deviation of the dens) and its ligamentous attachments
- May be a consequence of traumatic injury, particularly fracture of the dens
- Spinal cord trauma or compression at the junction between the atlas and axis—may cause neck pain and/or upper motor neuron tetraparesis to paralysis

SIGNALMENT
- Congenital—toy-breed dogs (poodles, Chihuahuas, Pekingese)
- Age at onset—usually before 12 months of age
- Uncommon in larger-breed dogs, dogs >1 year old, and cats
- No sex predilection

SIGNS
- Intermittent or progressive tetraparesis, usually with neck pain—most common
- Episodes of collapse—may occur
- May see proprioceptive deficits to complete paralysis, depending on degree of spinal cord compression or trauma
- Spinal reflexes—normal to exaggerated in all four limbs
- May lead to catastrophic acute spinal cord trauma, respiratory arrest, and death

CAUSES & RISK FACTORS
- Usually caused by abnormal formation of the dens
- Fracture of the dens

ATLANTOAXIAL INSTABILITY

- Clinical signs—may be exacerbated by activity, especially flexion of the neck
- Toy-breed dogs—at risk for congenital malformation of the dens

 DIAGNOSIS

DIFFERENTIAL DIAGNOSIS
- Disk herniation
- Fibrocartilaginous embolism
- Neoplasia
- Trauma
- Seizures
- With exercise intolerance—myasthenia gravis; hypoglycemia; hypoxia; cardiac abnormalities
- Diagnosis based on thorough physical examination and imaging

CBC/BIOCHEMISTRY/URINALYSIS
Normal

IMAGING
- Cervical spine radiographs—made with patient under general anesthesia; lateral view reveals increase in dorsal atlantoaxial space; lateral and ventrodorsal views reveal absence or fracture of dens.
- Hyperflex the neck only with extreme care during radiography; could cause severe spinal cord trauma and even death
- Myelography—seldom necessary for diagnosis

 TREATMENT

Conservative—reserved for patients with neck pain alone; includes neck brace and cage confinement for several weeks; recurrence common

Surgery
- Definitive; always indicated for neck pain with neurologic signs; dorsal and ventral approaches
- Dorsal approach—use wire or synthetic suture material to fix the dorsal spinous process of the axis to the dorsal arch of the atlas; common and serious postoperative complication: breakage of the dorsal arch of the atlas by the wire or suture
- Ventral approach—cancellous bone grafting and transarticular pinning; more stable; use polymethyl methacrylate to lock together the ventral tips of the pins to prevent pin migration; may use lag screws instead

 MEDICATIONS

DRUG(S)
Methylprednisolone sodium succinate—30 mg/kg; for acute paralysis and perioperatively

CONTRAINDICATIONS/POSSIBLE INTERACTIONS
- Glucocorticoids—use caution when given in conjunction with conservative treatment; may reduce pain, resulting in increased activity and spinal cord trauma
- Avoid NSAIDs in combination with glucocorticoids in all patients—increases risk of life-threatening gastrointestinal hemorrhage

 FOLLOW-UP

- Conservative treatment—re-evaluated weekly until clinical signs have resolved; often see recurrence, necessitating surgery
- Surgical treatment—usually no recurrent episodes; success influenced by the expertise and experience of the surgeon; intraoperative and immediately postoperative complications possible
- Untreated—may lead to catastrophic acute spinal cord trauma, respiratory arrest, and death

MISCELLANEOUS

Suggested Reading

Beaver DP, Ellison GW, Lewis DD. Risk factors affecting the outcome of surgery for atlantoaxial subluxation in dogs: 46 cases (1978–1998). J Am Vet Med Assoc 2000;216(7).

Fossum TW, Hedlund CS, Johnson AL, et al. Small animal surgery. St. Louis: Mosby–Year Book, 1997.

Shires PK. Atlantoaxial instability. In: Slatter D, ed. Textbook of small animal surgery. 3rd ed. Philadelphia: Saunders, 2003.

Acknowledgment

The author and editor acknowledge the prior contributions of Dr. Mary O. Smith.

Author: Peter K. Shires
Consulting Editor: Peter K. Shires

Craniomandibular Osteopathy

 BASICS

OVERVIEW
- A nonneoplastic, noninflammatory proliferative disease of the bones of the head
- Primary bones affected—mandibular rami; occipital and parietal; tympanic bullae; zygomatic portion of the temporal
- Bilateral symmetric involvement most common
- Affects musculoskeletal system

SIGNALMENT
- Scottish, cairn, and West Highland white terrier breeds—most common
- Labrador retrievers, Great Danes, Boston terriers, Doberman pinschers, Irish setters, English bulldogs, and boxers—may be affected
- Usually growing puppies 4–8 months of age
- No gender predilection
- Neutering may increase incidence.

SIGNS

Historical Findings
- Usually relate to pain around the mouth and difficulty eating
- Angular processes of the mandible affected—jaw movement progressively restricted
- Difficulty in prehension, mastication, and swallowing—may lead to starvation
- Lameness or limb swelling—may precede cranial involvement

Physical Examination Findings
- Temporal and masseter muscle atrophy—common
- Palpable irregular thickening of the mandibular rami and/or TMJ region

CRANIOMANDIBULAR OSTEOPATHY

- Inability to fully open jaw, even under general anesthesia
- Intermittent pyrexia—40°C
- Bilateral exophthalmos

CAUSES & RISK FACTORS
- Believed to be hereditary—occurs in certain breeds and families
- West Highland white terriers—autosomal recessive trait
- Scottish terriers—possible predisposition
- Possible link to infection—pyrexia; histologic evidence of inflammation only at the periphery of the lesion
- Young terrier with periosteal long bone disease—monitor for disease.

 DIAGNOSIS

DIFFERENTIAL DIAGNOSIS
- Osteomyelitis—bones not symmetrically affected; generally not as extensive; lysis; lack of breed predilection; history of penetrating wound
- Traumatic periostitis—bones not symmetrically affected; generally not as extensive; history of trauma
- Neoplasia—mature patient; not symmetrically affected; more lytic bone reaction; metastatic disease

CBC/BIOCHEMISTRY/URINALYSIS
- Serum ALP and inorganic phosphate—may be high
- May note hypogammaglobulinemia or α_2-hyperglobulinemia

OTHER LABORATORY TESTS
Serology—rule out fungal agents; indicated in atypical cases

IMAGING
- Skull radiography—reveals uneven, bead-like osseous proliferation of the mandible or tympanic bullae (bilateral); extensive, periosteal new bone formation (exostoses) affecting one or more bones around the TMJ; may show fusion of the tympanic bullae and angular process of the mandible
- CT—may help evaluate osseous involvement of the TMJ

DIAGNOSTIC PROCEDURES
Bone biopsy and culture (bacterial and fungal)—necessary only in atypical cases; rule out neoplasia and osteomyelitis

PATHOLOGIC FINDINGS
- Bone biopsy—reveals normal lamellar bone being replaced by an enlarged coarse-fiber bone and osteoclastic osteolysis of the periosteal or subperiosteal region
- Bone marrow—replaced by a vascular fibrous-type stroma
- Inflammatory cells—occasionally seen at the periphery of the bony lesion

 TREATMENT

- Palliative only
- Surgical excision of exostoses—results in regrowth within weeks
- High-calorie, protein-rich gruel diet—helps maintain nutritional balance
- Surgical placement of a pharyngostomy, esophagostomy, or gastrostomy tube—considered to help maintain nutritional balance

 MEDICATIONS

DRUG(S)
- Analgesics and antiinflammatory drugs—palliative use warranted
- NSAIDs—may be used to minimize pain and decrease inflammation; may try buffered or enteric-coated aspirin (10–25 mg/kg PO q8–12h), caroprofen (2.2 mg/kg PO q12h), etodolac (10–15 mg/kg, PO, once daily), phenylbutazone (3–7 mg/kg PO q8h, total dose < 800 mg/day), meclofenamic acid (0.5 mg/kg PO q12h), or piroxicam (0.3 mg/kg PO q24h for 3 days, then q48h)

CONTRAINDICATIONS/POSSIBLE INTERACTIONS
N/A

CRANIOMANDIBULAR OSTEOPATHY

 ## FOLLOW-UP

PATIENT MONITORING
Frequent re-examinations—mandatory to ensure adequate nutritional balance and pain control

PREVENTION/AVOIDANCE
- Do not repeat dam–sire breedings that resulted in affected offspring.
- Discourage breeding of affected animals.

EXPECTED COURSE AND PROGNOSIS
- Pain and discomfort may diminish at skeletal maturity (10–12 months of age); the exostoses may regress.
- Prognosis—depends on involvement of bones surrounding the TMJ
- Elective euthanasia may be necessary.

 ## MISCELLANEOUS

SYNONYMS
Lion jaw

ABBREVIATIONS
- ALP = alkaline phosphatase
- NSAIDS = nonsteroidal antiinflammatory drugs
- TMJ = temporomandibular joint

Suggested Reading
Watson ADJ, Adams WM, Thomas CB. Craniomandibular osteopathy in dogs. Compend Contin Educ Pract Vet 1995;17:911–921.

Author Peter D. Schwarz
Consulting Editor Peter K. Shires

Cruciate Ligament Disease, Cranial

 BASICS

DEFINITION
The acute or degenerative injury of the CrCL, which results in partial to complete instability of the stifle joint

PATHOPHYSIOLOGY
- Function of the CrCL—constrain the stifle joint by limiting internal rotation and cranial displacement of the tibia relative to the femur; prevents hyperextension
- CrCL injury—from trauma (acute) or degenerative causes (chronic); breaking strength approximately equal to four times the body weight of the dog
- Acute rupture—< 20% caused by exceeding the strength of the ligament in dogs; usually caused by hyperextension and excessive internal rotation with the stifle in partial flexion (20–50°); trauma most common cause in cats; a ligament weakened by degeneration is more easily ruptured than is a normal ligament.
- Degeneration—aging, conformational abnormalities, disuse related to sedentary habits or limb immobilization, and immune-mediated
- Aging and degeneration—related to size; dogs > 15 kg show more changes and have a more significant change in CrCL strength than do smaller dogs; degenerative changes and a decrease in material properties have been shown consistently in dogs > 5 years of age
- Conformational abnormalities—genu varum (bow-legged), genu valgum (knock-kneed), straight stifles and hock, caudal sloping of the tibial plateau, patella luxation, and narrowing of the intercondylar notch—may predispose patient to rupture.
- Immune-mediated arthritis, lymphocytic– plasmocytic synovitis, and septic arthritis—may predispose patient to rupture

CRUCIATE LIGAMENT DISEASE, CRANIAL

- Immune complexes—found in dogs with unilateral and bilateral rupture; unknown if they are a cause or a result of the rupture
- Partial rupture—accounts for 25–30% of stifle lameness cases
- Untreated rupture—degenerative changes within a few weeks; severe changes within a few months
- Medial meniscal (caudal horn) damage—from abnormal joint mechanics after CrCL injury; occurs in > 50% of cases
- Cranial tibial thrust—may play an important role in CrCL rupture; theoretically, a cranially directed force is generated during weight bearing, based on the caudal slope of the tibial plateau and the tibial compression mechanism

SYSTEMS AFFECTED
Musculoskeletal

GENETICS
- Unknown
- May be important in predisposing patient to DJD, degeneration of the CrCL, or conformation abnormalities

INCIDENCE/PREVALENCE
CrCL rupture—one of the most common causes of hindlimb lameness in dogs; major cause of DJD in the stifle joint

GEOGRAPHIC DISTRIBUTION
N/A

SIGNALMENT

Species
- Dogs
- Uncommon in cats

Breed Predilections
- All susceptible
- Rottweilers and Labrador retrievers—increased incidence of CrCL rupture when < 4 years of age

Mean Age and Range
- Dogs > 5 years of age
- Large breed dogs—between 1 and 2 years of age

Predominant Sex
Possibly female dogs

SIGNS

General Comments
Related to the degree of rupture (partial vs. complete), the mode of rupture (acute vs. chronic), the occurrence of meniscal injury, and the severity of inflammation and DJD

Historical Findings
- Athletic or traumatic events—generally precede acute injury, resulting in non-weight-bearing lameness with the affected limb held in flexion
- Normal activity resulting in acute lameness—suggests degenerative rupture
- Subtle to marked intermittent lameness (for weeks to months)—consistent with partial tears that are progressing to complete rupture

Physical Examination Findings
- Demonstration of cranial drawer motion—diagnostic for rupture; often dramatic after acute injury; subtle, almost imperceptible motion that ends gradually as a result of tissue stretching consistent with chronic rupture or partial tears; tested in flexion, normal standing angle, and extension
- Cranial movement of tibia relative to the femur during the tibial compression test
- Joint effusion
- Palpable thickening of the joint capsule—especially on the medial aspect (medial buttress)
- Hindlimb muscle atrophy—especially the quadriceps muscle group
- No cranial drawer sign (or negative tibial compression test)—does not rule out rupture; may see false-negative results with chronic or partial tears and in painful or anxious patients that are not sedated or anesthetized

CAUSES
- Trauma
- Degenerative changes

37

CRUCIATE LIGAMENT DISEASE, CRANIAL

- Conformation abnormalities
- Immune-mediated

RISK FACTORS
- Obesity
- Patella luxation
- Poor conformation
- Excessive caudal slope of tibial plateau
- Narrowed intercondylar notch

 DIAGNOSIS

DIFFERENTIAL DIAGNOSIS
- Skeletally immature dogs and dogs with significant muscle atrophy—slight drawer motion that stops abruptly as the CrCL is stretched taut is common
- Caudal cruciate ligament rupture—uncommon as an isolated occurrence
- Palpation—distinguish cranial from caudal rupture
- Patella luxation (medial or lateral)—alone or with CrCL rupture
- Stifle joint trauma
- Osteochondritis dissecans of the femoral condyle or patella
- Neoplasia (e.g., synovial cell sarcoma)—generally more painful than rupture

CBC/BIOCHEMISTRY/URINALYSIS
N/A

OTHER LABORATORY TESTS
N/A

IMAGING

Radiography
- Rarely diagnostic for rupture
- Extremely helpful in confirming intra-articular disease
- Common findings—joint effusion with capsular distention and compression of the infrapatellar fat pad; periarticular osteophytes; enthesiophytes; CrCL avulsion fractures; calcification of the CrCL

Magnetic Resonance Imaging
Graphically shows cruciate ligament and meniscal pathology

DIAGNOSTIC PROCEDURES
- Arthrocentesis—joint cytology to identify intra-articular disease and rule out sepsis and immune-mediated disease
- Arthroscopy—directly visualize the cruciate ligaments, menisci, and other intra-articular structures

PATHOLOGIC FINDINGS
- Varying degrees of cartilage fibrillation and erosion
- Periarticular osteophyte formation
- Meniscal damage
- Synovitis
- Ruptured fibers of the CrCL—hyalinization; fibrous tissue invasion; necrosis; loss of the parallel orientation of ligament bundles

 TREATMENT

APPROPRIATE HEALTH CARE
- Dogs < 15 kg—may treat conservatively as outpatients; 85% improve or are normal by 6 months
- Dogs > 15 kg—treated with surgery; only 20% improve or are normal by 6 months
- Surgery—recommended for all dogs; speeds rate of recovery; prevents degenerative changes; enhances function

NURSING CARE
Postsurgery—physical therapy (e.g., ice packing, range-of-motion exercises, massage, and muscle electrical stimulation); important for improving mobility and strength

ACTIVITY
Restricted—with conservative treatment and after surgical stabilization; duration depends on method of treatment and progress of patient.

DIET
Weight control—important for decreasing the load and thus stress on the stifle joint

CRUCIATE LIGAMENT DISEASE, CRANIAL

CLIENT EDUCATION
- Warn client that, regardless of the method of treatment, DJD is common.
- Inform client that return to complete athletic function is uncommon.
- Warn client that 20%–40% of dogs with unilateral CrCL rupture will experience rupture of the contralateral ligament within 17 months.

SURGICAL CONSIDERATIONS
No one technique has proven superior to the others.

Extra-articular Methods
- A wide variety of techniques that use a heavy-gauge implant to imbricate the joint and restore stability
- Implant material—placed in the approximate plane of the CrCL origin and insertion

Intra-articular Methods
- Designed to replace the CrCL anatomically
- Autografts (patella ligament, fascia), allografts (bone-tendon-bone), and synthetic materials—commonly used
- Femoral intercondylar notchplasty—recommended to minimize graft injury
- Arthroscopic replacement—recently described; long-term benefits unknown

Modified Extra-articular Methods
- Fibular head transposition or popliteal tendon transposition
- Realign and tension the lateral collateral ligament or popliteal tendon to restrict internal rotation and cranial drawer

Tibial Plateau Leveling Osteotomy
- Rotational osteotomy of the proximal tibia
- Levels tibial plateau and neutralizes cranial tibial thrust

 MEDICATIONS

DRUG(S) OF CHOICE
NSAIDs and analgesics—symptomatically treat associated synovitis and DJD; may use buffered or enteric-coated

aspirin (10–25 mg/kg PO q8–12h), caroprofen (2.2 mg/kg PO q12h), etodolac (10–15 mg/kg PO q24h), phenylbutazone (3–7 mg/kg PO q8h, total dose < 800 mg/day), meclofenamic acid (0.5 mg/kg PO q12h), piroxicam (0.3 mg/kg PO q24h for 3 days, then q48h), or deracoxib (3–4 mg/kg PO q24h for 7 days for postoperative pain) (1–2 mg/kg PO q24h for long-term treatment over 7 days)

CONTRAINDICATIONS
Avoid corticosteroids—potential side effects; articular cartilage damage associated with long-term use

PRECAUTIONS
NSAIDs—may cause gastrointestinal irritation; may preclude use in some patients

POSSIBLE INTERACTIONS
N/A

ALTERNATIVE DRUG(S)
Chondroprotective drugs (polysulfated glycosaminoglycans, glucosamine, and chondroitin sulfate)—may help limit cartilage damage and degeneration

 FOLLOW-UP

PATIENT MONITORING
- Depends on method of treatment
- Most techniques require 2–4 months of rehabilitation

PREVENTION/AVOIDANCE
Avoid breeding animals with conformation abnormalities.

POSSIBLE COMPLICATIONS
Second surgery—required in 10–15% of cases because of subsequent meniscal damage

EXPECTED COURSE AND PROGNOSIS
Regardless of surgical technique, the success rate is approximately 85%.

MISCELLANEOUS

ASSOCIATED CONDITIONS
Meniscal damage

AGE-RELATED FACTORS
See Pathophysiology

ZOONOTIC POTENTIAL
N/A

PREGNANCY
N/A

SEE ALSO
- Arthritis (Osteoarthritis)
- Patellar Luxation

ABBREVIATIONS
- CrCL = cranial cruciate ligament
- DJD = degenerative joint disease
- NSAID = nonsteroidal antiinflammatory drug

Suggested Reading

Brinker WO, Piermattei DL, Flo GL. Rupture of the cranial cruciate ligament. In: Brinker WO, Piermattei DL, Flo GL, eds. Handbook of small animal orthopedics and fracture repair. 3rd ed. Philadelphia: Saunders, 1997:534–563.

Johnson JM, Johnson AL. Cranial cruciate ligament rupture: pathogenesis, diagnosis, and postoperative rehabilitation. Vet Clin North Am 1993;23:717–733.

Slocum B, Slocum TD. Treatment of the stifle for cranial cruciate ligament rupture. In: Bojrab MJ, ed. Current techniques in small animal surgery. 4th ed. Philadelphia: Lea & Febiger, 1998:1187–1215.

Author: Peter D. Schwarz
Consulting Editor: Peter K. Shires

Diskospondylitis

BASICS

DEFINITION
A bacterial or fungal infection of the intervertebral disks and adjacent vertebral bodies

PATHOPHYSIOLOGY
- Hematogenous spread of bacterial or fungal organisms—most common cause
- Neurologic dysfunction—may occur; usually the result of spinal cord compression caused by proliferation of bone and fibrous tissue; less commonly owing to luxation or pathologic fracture of the spine, epidural abscess, or extension of infection to the meninges and spinal cord

SYSTEMS AFFECTED
- Musculoskeletal—infection and inflammation of the spine
- Nervous—compression of the spinal cord

GENETICS
- No definite predisposition identified
- An inherited immunodeficiency has been detected in a few cases.

INCIDENCE/PREVALENCE
Approximately 0.2% of dog hospital admissions

GEOGRAPHIC DISTRIBUTION
Grass awn migration and coccidiomycosis—more common in certain regions

SIGNALMENT

Species
Dogs; rare in cats

Breed Predilection
Large and giant breeds, especially German shepherds and Great Danes

43

DISKOSPONDYLITIS

Mean Age and Range
- Mean age —4–5 years
- Range—5 months to 12 years

Predominant Sex
Males outnumber females by ~2:1

SIGNS

Historical Findings
- Onset usually relatively acute; some patients have mild signs for several months before examination.
- Pain—difficulty rising, reluctance to jump, and stilted gait are most common signs.
- Ataxia or paresis
- Weight loss and anorexia
- Lameness
- Draining tracts

Physical Examination Findings
- Focal or multifocal areas of spinal pain in >80% of patients
- Any disk space may be affected; lumbosacral space is most commonly involved.
- Paresis or paralysis, especially in chronic, untreated cases
- Fever in ~30% of patients
- Lameness

CAUSES
- Bacterial—*Staphylococcus intermedius* is the most common. Others include *Streptococcus, Brucella canis,* and *E. coli,* but virtually any bacteria can be causative.
- Fungal—*Aspergillus, Paecilomyces,* and *Coccidioides immitis*
- Grass awn migration is often associated with mixed infections, especially *Actinomyces;* tends to affect the L2–L4 disk spaces and vertebrae
- Other causes—surgery, bite wounds

RISK FACTORS
- Urinary tract infection
- Periodontal disease
- Bacterial endocarditis

- Dermatitis
- Immunodeficiency

 DIAGNOSIS

DIFFERENTIAL DIAGNOSIS
- Intervertebral disk protrusion—may cause similar clinical signs; differentiated on the basis of radiography and myelography
- Vertebral fracture or luxation—detected on radiographs
- Vertebral neoplasia—usually does not affect adjacent vertebral end plates
- Spondylosis deformans—rarely causes clinical signs; has similar radiographic features, including sclerosis, ventral spur formation, and collapse of the disk space; rarely causes lysis of the vertebral end plates
- Focal meningomyelitis—often identified by CSF analysis

CBC/BIOCHEMISTRY/URINALYSIS
- Hemogram—often normal; may see leukocytosis
- Urinalysis—may reveal pyuria and/or bacteriuria with concurrent urinary tract infections

OTHER LABORATORY TESTS
- Aerobic, anaerobic, and fungal blood cultures identify the causative organism in up to 75% of cases; obtain if available.
- Sensitivity testing—indicated if cultures are positive
- Urine cultures—indicated; positive in about 25% of patients
- Organisms other than *Staphylococcus* spp.—may not be the cause
- Serologic testing for *Brucella canis*—indicated

IMAGING
- Spinal radiography—usually reveals lysis of vertebral end plates adjacent to the affected disk, collapse of the disk space, and varying degrees of sclerosis of the end plates and ventral spur formation; may not see lesions until 3–4 weeks after infection

DISKOSPONDYLITIS

- Myelography—indicated with substantial neurologic deficits; determine location and degree of spinal cord compression, especially if considering decompressive surgery; spinal cord compression caused by diskospondylitis typically displays an extradural pattern.
- Computed tomography or magnetic resonance imaging—more sensitive than radiography; indicated when radiographs are normal or inconclusive

DIAGNOSTIC PROCEDURES
- CSF analysis—occasionally indicated to rule out meningomyelitis; usually normal or reveals mildly high protein
- Bone scintigraphy—occasionally useful for detecting early lesions; helps clarify if radiographic changes are infectious or degenerative (spondylosis deformans)
- Fluoroscopically guided fine-needle aspiration of the disk—valuable for obtaining tissue for culture when blood and urine cultures are negative and there is no improvement with empiric antibiotic therapy

PATHOLOGIC FINDINGS
- Gross—loss of normal disk space; bony proliferation of adjacent vertebrae
- Microscopic—fibrosing pyogranulomatous destruction of the disk and vertebral bodies

 TREATMENT

APPROPRIATE HEALTH CARE
- Outpatient—mild pain
- Inpatient—severe pain or progressive neurologic deficits

NURSING CARE
Nonambulatory patients—keep on a clean, dry, well-padded surface to prevent decubitus ulcers.

ACTIVITY
Restricted

DIET
Normal

CLIENT EDUCATION
- Explain that observation of response to treatment is very important in determining the need for further diagnostic or therapeutic procedures.
- Instruct the client to immediately contact the veterinarian if clinical signs progress or recur or if neurologic deficits develop.

SURGICAL CONSIDERATIONS
- Curettage of a single affected disk space—occasionally necessary for patients that are refractory to antibiotic therapy
- Goals—remove infected tissue; obtain tissue for culture and histologic evaluation
- Decompression of the spinal cord by hemilaminectomy or dorsal laminectomy—indicated for substantial neurologic deficits and spinal cord compression evident on myelography when there is no improvement with antibiotic therapy; also perform curettage of the infected disk space; it may be necessary to perform surgical stabilization if more than one articular facet is removed.

 MEDICATIONS

DRUGS OF CHOICE

Antibiotics
- Selection based on results of blood cultures and serology
- Negative culture and serology—assume causative organism is Staphylococcus spp.; treat with a cephalosporin (e.g., cefadroxil; dogs: 22 mg/kg PO q12h; cats: 22 mg/kg PO q24h).
- Acutely progressive signs or substantial neurologic deficits—initially treated with parenteral antibiotics (e.g., cefazolin; dogs and cats: 20–35 mg/kg IV q8h); continued for at least 6 weeks
- Brucellosis—treated with tetracycline (dogs: 15 mg/kg PO q8h) and streptomycin (dogs: 3.4 mg/kg IM q24h) or enrofloxacin (dogs: 2.5–5.0 mg/kg PO q12h)

DISKOSPONDYLITIS

Analgesics
- Signs of severe pain—treated with an analgesic (e.g., oxymorphone; dogs: 0.05–0.2 mg/kg IV, IM, SC q4–6h)
- Taper dosage after 3–5 days to gauge effectiveness of antibiotic therapy.

CONTRAINDICATIONS
Glucocorticoids

PRECAUTIONS
Use NSAIDs and other analgesics cautiously—may cause a temporary resolution of clinical signs even when infection is progressing; when used, discontinue after 3–5 days to assess efficacy of antibiotic therapy.

POSSIBLE INTERACTIONS
None

ALTERNATIVE DRUGS
- Initial therapy—cephradine (dogs: 20 mg/kg PO q8h); cloxacillin (dogs: 10 mg/kg PO q8h)
- Refractory patients—clindamycin (dogs and cats: 10 mg/kg PO q12h), enrofloxacin (dogs: 5–20 mg/kg PO q24h; cats: 5 mg/kg PO q24h), orbifloxacin (dogs and cats: 2.5–7.5 mg/kg PO q24h)

 FOLLOW-UP

PATIENT MONITORING
- Reevaluate after 5 days of therapy
- No improvement in pain, fever, or appetite—reassess therapy; consider a different antibiotic, percutaneous aspiration of the affected disk space, or surgery.
- Improvement—evaluate clinically and radiographically every 2–4 weeks.

PREVENTION/AVOIDANCE
Early identification of predisposing causes and prompt diagnosis and treatment—help reduce progression of clinical symptoms and neurologic deterioration

POSSIBLE COMPLICATIONS
- Spinal cord compression owing to proliferative bony and fibrous tissue
- Vertebral fracture or luxation
- Meningitis or meningomyelitis
- Epidural abscess

EXPECTED COURSE AND PROGNOSIS
- Recurrence is common if antibiotic therapy is stopped prematurely (before 6 weeks of treatment).
- Prognosis—depends on causative organism and degree of spinal cord damage
- Mild or no neurologic dysfunction (dogs)—usually respond within 5 days of starting antibiotic therapy
- Substantial paresis or paralysis (dogs)—prognosis guarded; may note gradual resolution of neurologic dysfunction after several weeks of therapy; treatment warranted
- *Brucella canis*—signs usually resolve with therapy; infection may not be eradicated; recurrence common

 MISCELLANEOUS

ASSOCIATED CONDITIONS
See Risk Factors.

AGE-RELATED FACTORS
N/A

ZOONOTIC POTENTIAL
Brucella canis—human infection uncommon but may occur

PREGNANCY
N/A

SYNONYMS
- Intradiskal osteomyelitis
- Intervertebral disk infection
- Vertebral osteomyelitis
- Diskitis

DISKOSPONDYLITIS

SEE ALSO
Brucellosis

ABBREVIATION
CSF = cerebrospinal fluid

Suggested Reading

Davis MJ, Dewey CW, Walker MA, et al. Contrast radiographic findings in canine bacterial discospondylitis: A multicenter, retrospective study of 27 cases. J Am Anim Hosp Assoc 2000;36:81–85

Fischer A, Mahaffey MB, Oliver JE. Fluoroscopically guided percutaneous disk aspiration in 10 dogs with diskospondylitis. J Vet Intern Med 1997;11:284–287.

Johnson RG, Prata RG. Intradiskal osteomyelitis: a conservative approach. J Am Anim Hosp Assoc 1983;19:743–750.

Kerwin SC, Lewis DD, Hribernik TN, et al. Diskospondylitis associated with Brucella canis infection in dogs: 14 cases (1989–1991). J Am Vet Med Assoc 1992;201:1253–1257.

Kornegay JN. Diskospondylitis. In: Kirk RW, ed. Current veterinary therapy IX. Philadelphia: Saunders, 1986:810–814.

Thomas WB. Diskospondylitis and other vertebral infections. Vet Clin North Am Small Anim Pract 2000;30:169–182.

Author: William B. Thomas
Consulting Editor: Peter K. Shires

Elbow Dysplasia

 BASICS

DEFINITION
A series of four developmental abnormalities that lead to malformation and degeneration of the elbow joint

PATHOPHYSIOLOGY
- Four abnormalities—UAP, OCD, FMCP, and incongruity; may occur alone or in combination; may be seen in one or both elbows; bilateral disease common (50% of cases)
- UAP—characterized by failure of the anconeal process (which contains a separate ossification center) to unite with the proximal ulnar metaphysis (olecranon) by 5 months of age; may be the result of abnormal mechanical stress on the anconeal process
- OCD—affects the medial aspect of the humeral condyle; retention of articular cartilage due to a disturbance in endochondral ossification and mechanical stress; leads to formation of a cartilage flap lesion; may be the result of abnormal mechanical stress on the medial aspect
- FMCP—chondral or osteochondral fragmentation or fissure of the medial coronoid process of the ulna; not considered a traumatic injury; a manifestation of osteo-chondrosis of the coronoid process; differs from the related pathology of the anconeal process because the coronoid does not have a separate ossification center; may be the result of abnormal mechanical stress on the medial coronoid process
- Incongruity—manifestation of malalignment and malformation of the elbow joint; asynchronous proximal growth between the radius and ulna may lead to abnormal load and to wear and erosion of cartilage in the humeroulnar compartment; may be the result of malfor-mation of the trochlear notch of the ulna; a slightly ellipti-cal trochlear notch with a decreased arc of curvature is

ELBOW DYSPLASIA

too small to articulate with the humeral trochlea, which results in major points of contact in areas of the anconeal process, coronoid process, and medial humeral condyle and little or no contact in other areas of the trochlea

SYSTEMS AFFECTED
Musculoskeletal

GENETICS
- Inherited disease
- High heritability—heritability index ranges between 0.25 and 0.45.

INCIDENCE/PREVALENCE
- Most common cause for elbow pain and lameness
- One of the most common causes for forelimb lameness in large-breed dogs

GEOGRAPHIC DISTRIBUTION
N/A

SIGNALMENT

Species
Dogs

Breed Predilections
Large and giant breeds—Labrador retrievers; Rottweilers; golden retrievers; German shepherds; Bernese mountain dogs; chow chows; bearded collies; Newfoundlands

Mean Age and Range
- Age at onset of clinical signs—typically 4–10 months
- Age at diagnosis—generally 4–18 months
- Onset of symptoms related to DJD—any age

Predominant Sex
- FMCP—males predisposed
- UAP, OCD, incongruity—none established

SIGNS

General Comments
- Lameness—if no distinct abnormalities noted on physical examination or radiographs, repeat examination 4–8 weeks later.

- Not all patients are symptomatic when young.
- Acute episode of elbow lameness due to advanced DJD changes in a mature patient—common

Historical Findings
Intermittent or persistent forelimb lameness—exacerbated by exercise; progressed from a stiffness seen only after rest

Physical Examination Findings
- Pain—elicited on elbow hyperflexion or extension; elicited when holding the elbow and carpus at 90° while pronating and supinating the carpus
- Affected limb—tendency to be held in abduction and supination
- Joint effusion and capsular distension—especially noted between the lateral epicondyle and olecranon
- Crepitus—may be palpated with advanced DJD
- Diminished range of motion

CAUSES
- Genetic
- Developmental
- Nutritional

RISK FACTORS
- Rapid growth and weight gain
- High-calorie diet

 DIAGNOSIS

DIFFERENTIAL DIAGNOSIS
- Trauma
- Septic arthritis
- Panosteitis
- Avulsion or calcification of the flexor muscles
- Synovial cell sarcoma

CBC/BIOCHEMISTRY/URINALYSIS
N/A

OTHER LABORATORY TESTS
N/A

ELBOW DYSPLASIA

IMAGING

Radiography
- May need four views for diagnosis—mediolateral; mediolateral hyperflexed; 25° craniocaudal-lateromedial oblique; craniocaudal
- Image both elbows—high incidence of bilateral disease
- UAP—best diagnosed from the mediolateral hyperflexed view; may easily see lack of bony union
- OCD—best diagnosed from the craniocaudal and craniocaudal-lateromedial oblique views; reveals a radiolucent defect or flattening of the medial aspect of the humeral condyle
- FMCP—seldom visualized; diagnosis is presumptive based on DJD and the absence of UAP or OCD lesions; commonly see osteophyte formation on the proximal rim of the anconeal process, medial coronoid process, and cranial margin of the radial head and epicondyles (medial and lateral); also commonly see sclerosis of the ulna caudal to the coronoid process and trochlear notch and stairstep between the joint surface of the radius and lateral coronoid; may also see these changes with UAP, OCD, and incongruity

Other
CT, MRI, and linear tomography—accurately diagnose FMCP

DIAGNOSTIC PROCEDURES
- Joint tap and analysis of synovial fluid—confirm involvement of joint
- Synovial fluid—should be straw colored with normal to decreased viscosity; cytology reveals < 10,000 nucleated cells/μL (> 90% are mononuclear cells); normal results do not necessarily rule out the diagnosis.
- Arthroscopy—may use to diagnose UAP, FMCP, and OCD

PATHOLOGIC FINDINGS
- UAP—fibrous union between anconeal process and proximal ulnar metaphysis; fibrous tissue invasion and degeneration of the anconeal process; DJD

- OCD—chondral flap on medial humeral condyle; sclerosis of underlying subchondral bone with fibrous tissue invasion; erosive lesion on apposing coronoid cartilage; DJD
- FMCP—chondral or osteochondral fragmentation of the cranial tip or lateral margin of the medial coronoid; erosive lesion on cartilage of the apposing medial aspect of the humeral condyle; DJD
- Incongruity—erosive lesions involving part or all of medial coronoid process and the apposing articular cartilage of the medial aspect of the humeral condyle; DJD; linear striations in the articular cartilage

 TREATMENT

APPROPRIATE HEALTH CARE
Surgery—controversial but recommended for all patients

NURSING CARE
- Cold packing the elbow joint—perform immediately postsurgery to help decrease swelling and control pain; perform at least 15–20 min q8h for 3–5 days.
- Range-of-motion exercises—beneficial until the patient can bear weight on the limb(s)

ACTIVITY
Restricted for all patients postoperatively

DIET
- Weight control—important for decreasing the load and stress on the affected joint(s)
- Restricted weight gain and growth in young dogs—may decrease incidence and severity

CLIENT EDUCATION
- Discuss the heritability of the disease.
- Discuss the potential for DJD progression.
- Discuss the influence of excessive intake of nutrients that promote rapid growth.

SURGICAL CONSIDERATIONS
- Severity of DJD and age of patient—negatively influence outcome

ELBOW DYSPLASIA

- UAP—four options: removal, lag screw fixation, dynamic proximal ulnar osteotomy, and lag screw fixation plus dynamic proximal osteotomy; base decision on degree of DJD, patient's age, and surgical expertise.
- OCD and FMCP—medial approach to elbow (diagnostic differentiation not necessary); removal of loose fragment(s)
- Incongruity—controversial; four options: no surgery, coronoidectomy, dynamic proximal ulnar osteotomy, intra-articular osteotomy; base decision on type of incongruity, degree of DJD, patient's age, and surgical expertise.
- Arthroscopic diagnosis and treatment—excellent option for FMCP, OCD, and incongruity; benefits: superior diagnostic capabilities, minimal invasiveness, decreased postoperative discomfort, and decreased postoperative morbidity

 MEDICATIONS

DRUG(S) OF CHOICE
- None that promotes healing of osteochondral or chondral fragments
- NSAIDs—minimize pain, decrease inflammation, symptomatically treat associated DJD; may try buffered or enteric-coated aspirin (10–25 mg/kg PO q8–12h), caroprofen (2.2 mg/kg PO q12h), etodolac (10–15 mg/kg PO q24h), phenylbutazone (3–7 mg/kg PO q8h, dose < 800 mg/day), meclofenamic acid (0.5 mg/kg PO q12h), and piroxicam (0.3 mg/kg PO q24h for 3 days then q48h), deracoxib (3–4 mg/kg PO q24h for 7 days for postoperative pain) (1–2 mg/kg PO q24h for long-term treatment over 7 days)

CONTRAINDICATIONS
Avoid corticosteroids—potential side effects; articular carti-lage damage associated with long-term use

PRECAUTIONS
NSAIDs—gastrointestinal irritation may preclude use in some patients.

POSSIBLE INTERACTIONS
N/A

ALTERNATIVE DRUG(S)
Chondroprotective drugs (e.g., polysulfated glycosaminogly-cans, glucosamine, and chondroitin sulfate)—may help limit cartilage damage and degeneration; may help alleviate pain and inflammation

 FOLLOW-UP

PATIENT MONITORING
- Postsurgery—limit activity for a minimum of 4 weeks; encourage early, active movement of the affected joint(s).
- Yearly examinations—recommended to evaluate progression of DJD

PREVENTION/AVOIDANCE
- Discourage breeding of affected animals.
- Do not repeat dam–sire breedings that result in affected offspring.

POSSIBLE COMPLICATIONS
N/A

EXPECTED COURSE AND PROGNOSIS
- Progression of DJD—expected
- Prognosis—fair to good for all forms

 MISCELLANEOUS

ASSOCIATED CONDITIONS
N/A

AGE-RELATED FACTORS
Middle-aged to old dogs with advanced DJD are not candidates for surgical intervention.

ZOONOTIC POTENTIAL
N/A

PREGNANCY
N/A

ELBOW DYSPLASIA

SYNONYMS
Elbow osteochondrosis

SEE ALSO
Osteochondrosis

ABBREVIATIONS
- CT = computed tomography
- DJD = degenerative joint disease
- FMCP = fragmented medial coronoid process
- MRI = magnetic resonance imaging
- NSAIDs = nonsteroidal antiinflammatory drugs
- OCD = osteochondritis dissecans
- UAP = un-united anconeal process

Suggested Reading

Olsson SE. Pathophysiology, morphology, and clinical signs of osteochondrosis in the dog. In: Bojrab MJ, ed. Disease mechanisms in small animal surgery. Philadelphia: Lea & Febiger, 1993:777–779.

Schwarz PD. Elbow dysplasia. In: Bonagura JD, Kersey R, eds. Current veterinary therapy XIII: Small animal practice. Philadelphia: Saunders, 2000:1004–1014.

Wind AP. Elbow incongruity and developmental elbow diseases in the dog: parts I and II. J Am Anim Hosp Assoc 1986; 22:711–724.

Author Peter D. Schwarz
Consulting Editor Peter K. Shires

Hip Dysplasia–Dogs

 BASICS

DEFINITION
The malformation and degeneration of the coxofemoral joints

PATHOPHYSIOLOGY
- Developmental defect initiated by a genetic predisposition to subluxation of the immature hip joint
- Poor congruence between the femoral head and acetabulum—creates abnormal forces across the joint; interferes with normal development (leading to irregularly shaped acetabula and femoral heads); overloads the articular cartilage (causing microfractures and DJD)

SYSTEMS AFFECTED
Musculoskeletal

GENETICS
- Complicated, polygenetic transmission
- Expression—determined by an interaction of genetic and environmental factors
- Heritability index—depends on breed

INCIDENCE/PREVALENCE
- One of the most common skeletal diseases encountered clinically in dogs
- Actual incidence—unknown; depends on breed

GEOGRAPHIC DISTRIBUTION
N/A

SIGNALMENT

Species
Dogs

Breed Predilection
- Large breeds—St. Bernards; German shepherds; Labrador retrievers; golden retrievers; rottweilers

HIP DYSPLASIA—DOGS

- Smaller breeds—may be affected; less likely to demonstrate clinical signs

Mean Age and Range
- Begins in the immature dog
- Clinical signs—may develop after 4 months of age; may develop later with DJD

Predominant Sex
None

SIGNS

General Comments
- Depend on the degree of joint laxity, degree of DJD, and chronicity of the disease
- Early—related to joint laxity
- Later—related to joint degeneration

Historical Findings
- Decreased activity
- Difficulty rising
- Reluctance to run, jump, or climb stairs
- Intermittent or persistent hind limb lameness—often worse after exercise
- Bunny-hopping or swaying gait
- Narrow stance in the hind limbs

Physical Examination Findings
- Pain
- Joint laxity (positive Ortolani sign)—characteristic of early disease; may not be seen in chronic cases owing to periarticular fibrosis
- Crepitus
- Decreased range of motion in the hip joints
- Atrophy of thigh muscles
- Hypertrophy of shoulder muscles

CAUSES
- Genetic predisposition for hip laxity
- Rapid weight gain, nutrition level, and pelvic muscle mass—influence expression and progression

RISK FACTORS
N/A

DIAGNOSIS

DIFFERENTIAL DIAGNOSIS
- Degenerative myelopathy
- Lumbosacral instability
- Bilateral stifle disease
- Panosteitis
- Polyarthropathies

CBC/BIOCHEMISTRY/URINALYSIS
N/A

OTHER LABORATORY TESTS
N/A

IMAGING
- Ventrodorsal hip-extended radiographs—commonly used for diagnosis; may need sedation or general anesthesia for accurate positioning
- Early radiographic signs—subluxation of the hip joint with poor congruence between the femoral head and acetabulum; initially normally shaped acetabulum and femoral head; with disease progression, shallow acetabulum, and flattened femoral head
- Radiographic evidence of DJD—flattening of the femoral head; shallow acetabulum; periarticular osteophyte production; thickening of the femoral neck; sclerosis of the subchondral bone; periarticular soft tissue fibrosis
- Distraction radiographs—quantify joint laxity; may accentuate the laxity for more accurate diagnosis
- PennHIP registry uses distraction radiography method. Dorsolateral subluxation (DLS) is another available distraction radiography method.
- Dorsal acetabular rim view radiographs—evaluate acetabular rim; assess dorsal coverage of the femoral head

DIAGNOSTIC PROCEDURES
N/A

PATHOLOGIC FINDINGS
- Early—normal femoral head and acetabulum; may note joint laxity and excess synovial fluid

HIP DYSPLASIA—DOGS

- With progression—malformed acetabulum and femoral head; synovitis; articular cartilage degeneration
- Chronic—may note full-thickness cartilage erosion

 TREATMENT

APPROPRIATE HEALTH CARE
- May treat with conservative medical therapy or surgery
- Outpatient unless surgery is performed
- Depends on the patient's size, age, and intended function; severity of joint laxity; degree of DJD; clinician's preference; and financial considerations of the owner

NURSING CARE
- Physiotherapy (passive joint motion)—decreases joint stiffness; helps maintain muscle integrity
- Swimming (hydrotherapy)—excellent nonconcussive form of physical therapy; encourages joint and muscle activity without exacerbating joint injury

ACTIVITY
- As tolerated
- Swimming—recommended to maintain joint mobility while minimizing weight-bearing activities

DIET
Weight control—important; decrease the load applied to the painful joint; minimize weight gain associated with reduced exercise

CLIENT EDUCATION
- Discuss the heritability of the disease.
- Explain that medical therapy is palliative, because the joint instability is not corrected.
- Warn the client that joint degeneration often progresses unless a corrective osteotomy procedure is performed early in the disease.
- Explain that surgical procedures can salvage joint function once severe joint degeneration occurs.

SURGICAL CONSIDERATIONS

Triple Pelvic Osteotomy

- Corrective procedure; designed to reestablish congruity between the femoral head and the acetabulum
- Immature patient (6–12 months of age)
- Rotate acetabulum—improve dorsal coverage of the femoral head; correct the forces acting on the joint; minimize the progression of DJD; may allow development of a more normal joint if performed early (before severe degeneration develops)

Juvenile Pubic Symphysiodesis

- Newly developed technique still under evaluation
- Pubic symphysis is fused at an early age (using electrocautery).
- Causes ventroversion of the acetabulum to better cover the femoral head
- Improves joint congruence and stability—similar effects as TPO without surgical implants
- Minimal morbidity; easy to perform—must be performed very early (3–4 months of age) to achieve effect; minimal effect achieved if performed after 6 months of age

Total Hip Replacement

- Indicated to salvage function in mature dogs with severe degenerative disease that is unresponsive to medical therapy
- Pain-free joint function—reported in >90% of cases
- Unilateral joint replacement—provides acceptable function in ~80% of cases
- Complications—luxation; sciatic neuropraxia; infection

Excision Arthroplasty

- Removal of the femoral head and neck to eliminate joint pain
- Primarily a salvage procedure—for significant DJD; when pain cannot be controlled medically; when total hip replacement is cost-prohibitive
- Best results—small, light dogs (< 20 kg); patients with good hip musculature

63

HIP DYSPLASIA—DOGS

- A slightly abnormal gait often persists.
- Postoperative muscle atrophy—common, particularly in large dogs

 MEDICATIONS

DRUG(S) OF CHOICE
- Analgesics and anti-inflammatory drugs—minimize joint pain (and thus stiffness and muscle atrophy caused by limited usage); decrease synovitis
- Medical therapy—does not correct biomechanical abnormality; degenerative process likely to progress; often provides only temporary relief of signs
- Agents—carprofen (2.2 mg/kg PO q12h or 4.4 mg/kg PO q24h); etodolac (10–15 mg/kg PO q24h); deracoxib (3–4 mg/kg PO q24h for 1 week for postoperative pain) (1–2 mg/kg PO q24h for long-term treatment over 7 days)

CONTRAINDICATIONS
Avoid corticosteroids—potential side effects; articular cartilage damage associated with long-term use

PRECAUTIONS
- NSAIDs—gastrointestinal upset may preclude use in some patients.
- Carprofen—reported to cause acute hepatotoxicity in some dogs

POSSIBLE INTERACTIONS
N/A

ALTERNATIVE DRUG(S)
Polysulfated glycosaminoglycans, glucosamine, and chondroitin sulfate—may have a chondroprotective effect in DJD; not fully evaluated for treatment of hip dysplasia

FOLLOW-UP

PATIENT MONITORING
- Clinical and radiographic monitoring—assess progression.
- Medical treatment—clinical deterioration suggests an alternative dosage or medication or surgical intervention.
- Triple pelvic osteotomy—monitored radiographically; assess healing, implant stability, joint congruence, and progression of DJD.
- Hip replacement—monitored radiographically; assess implant stability.

PREVENTION/AVOIDANCE
- Best prevented by not breeding affected dogs
- Pelvic radiographs—may help identify phenotypically abnormal dogs; may not identify all dogs carrying the disease
- Do not repeat dam–sire breedings that result in affected offspring.
- Special diets designed for rapidly growing large-breed dogs—may decrease the severity

POSSIBLE COMPLICATIONS
N/A

EXPECTED COURSE AND PROGNOSIS
Joint degeneration usually progresses—most patients lead normal lives with proper medical or surgical management.

 MISCELLANEOUS

ASSOCIATED CONDITIONS
N/A

AGE-RELATED FACTORS
N/A

ZOONOTIC POTENTIAL
N/A

HIP DYSPLASIA–DOGS

PREGNANCY

Do not breed affected dogs; added weight owing to pregnancy may exacerbate clinical signs.

ABBREVIATIONS

DJD = degenerative joint disease
TPO = triple pelvic osteotomy
NSAIDs = nonsteroidal antiinflammatory drugs

Suggested Reading

Manley PA. The hip joint. In: Slatter D, ed. Textbook of small animal surgery. 2nd ed. Philadelphia: Saunders, 1993:1786–1804.

McLaughlin RM, Tomlinson J. Alternative surgical treatments for canine hip dysplasia. Vet Med 1996;91:137–143.

McLaughlin RM, Tomlinson J. Radiographic diagnosis of canine hip dysplasia. Vet Med 1996;91:36–47.

McLaughlin RM, Tomlinson J. Treating canine hip dysplasia with triple pelvic osteotomy. Vet Med 1996;91:126–136.

Rettenmaier JL, Constantinescu GM. Canine hip dysplasia. Compend Contin Educ Pract Vet 1991;13:643–653.

Swainson SW, Conzemius MG, Riedesel EA, Smith GK, Riley CB. Effect of pubic symphysiodesis on pelvic development in the skeletally immature greyhound. Vet Surg 29:178–190, 2000.

Tomlinson J, McLaughlin RM. Canine hip dysplasia: developmental factors, clinical signs and initial examination steps. Vet Med 1996;91:26–33.

Tomlinson J, McLaughlin RM. Medically managing canine hip dysplasia. Vet Med 1996;91:48–53.

Tomlinson J, McLaughlin RM. Total hip replacement. Vet Med 1996;91:118–124.

Wallace LJ. Canine hip dysplasia: past and present. Semin Vet Med Surg 1987;2:92–106.

Author: Ron M. McLaughlin
Consulting Editor: Peter K. Shires

Hypertrophic Osteodystrophy

 BASICS

DEFINITION
An inflammatory disease of bone that affects rapidly growing puppies

PATHOPHYSIOLOGY
- Characterized by nonseptic suppurative inflammation within metaphyseal trabeculae of long bones
- Rapidly growing bones more severely affected
- Metaphyses—widened owing to perimetaphyseal swelling and bone deposition
- Trabecular microfracture and metaphyseal separation—occur adjacent and parallel to the physis
- Bone formation defective
- Ossifying periostitis—may be extensive

SYSTEMS AFFECTED
- Musculoskeletal—symmetrical distribution; distal forelimbs most severely affected; may note soft tissue mineralization in other organs; widened costochondral junctions
- Respiratory—interstitial pneumonia
- Gastrointestinal—diarrhea

GENETICS
No basis

INCIDENCE/PREVALENCE
Low

GEOGRAPHIC DISTRIBUTION
N/A

SIGNALMENT

Species
Dogs

HYPERTROPHIC OSTEODYSTROPHY

Breed Predilections
- Large, rapidly growing breeds
- Great Danes—most common
- Reported—Irish wolfhounds; St. Bernards; Kuvasz; Irish setters; Weimaraners; Doberman pinschers; German shepherds; Labrador retrievers; many others

Mean Age and Range
- Affects only growing puppies
- Mean—3–4 months
- Range of onset—2–8 months

Predominant Sex
Males more than females

SIGNS

General Comments
Lameness—may be episodic; degree varies from mild to non–weight-bearing; initial episode may resolve without relapse.

Historical Findings
- Depend on severity of the episode
- Owners often describe a depressed puppy that is reluctant to move.
- Inappetence—common

Physical Examination Findings
- Lameness—symmetrical, more severe in forelimbs
- Metaphyses—painful; warm; swollen
- Pyrexia—as high as 41.1°C (106°F)
- Inappetence
- Depression
- Weight loss
- Dehydration
- Diarrhea
- Cachexia
- Debilitation
- Manifestations of systemic illness—respiratory or gastrointestinal

CAUSES
Unknown; the following hypotheses have been proposed.

Metabolic

- Hypovitaminosis C—discounted; many patients have normal ascorbic acid values; supplementation does not resolve disease or prevent relapses; dogs synthesize their own vitamin C; histologic changes differ from those of disease.
- Hypocuprosis—produces histologic changes in rats similar to those seen in affected puppies; does not cause similar changes in dogs

Nutritional

- Overnutrition and oversupplementation—association inconsistent at best
- Only one or two affected puppies within a litter; however, all receive the same diet and supplementation.
- Has occurred in puppies that were not overfed or oversupplemented
- Correcting diet does not alter the course of the disease or eliminate relapses.

Infectious

- Bacterial or fungal organisms—not identified histopathologically in tissues from affected puppies
- Unable to transmit the disease hematogenously from affected to unaffected puppies
- Canine distemper virus RNA—detected in bone cells of patients; unaffected dogs injected with blood from patients developed distemper (3 of 7 dogs) but not hypertrophic osteodystrophy.
- Secondary development may depend on the timing of the neonate's exposure.

RISK FACTORS
None proven

 DIAGNOSIS

DIFFERENTIAL DIAGNOSIS

- Juvenile bone and joint disorders
- Panosteitis—no metaphyseal swelling; cottony intramedullary densities in long bones on radiographs

HYPERTROPHIC OSTEODYSTROPHY

- Elbow dysplasia—no metaphyseal swelling; no fever; pain localized to the elbow(s); typical radiographic signs
- Osteochondritis dissecans—no metaphyseal swelling or fever; pain localized to shoulder or elbow; subchondral defects on radiographs
- Septic polyarthritis—swelling more localized to joint capsule; soft tissue swelling localized to the joint on radiographs; septic suppurative inflammation on arthrocentesis; culture
- Nonseptic polyarthritis—nonseptic suppurative inflammation on arthrocentesis; direct diagnostics toward other causes (e.g., *Ehrlichia canis*)
- Septic metaphysitis—radiographs of the extremities not typical of hypertrophic osteodystrophy; asymmetrical; may note septic suppurative inflammation on needle aspiration of metaphyseal lesions; hematologic findings implicate bacterial infection (neutrophilia with accompanying left shift).
- Retained cartilage cores—young large and giant breeds; valgus deformity of the distal forelimbs caused by retained cartilage core in the distal ulnar physes; retained cartilage on radiographs; afebrile; less perimetaphyseal swelling; less or no pain with manipulation
- Canine osteochondrodysplasias—developmental disorders; various breeds; cartilage abnormalities and abnormal bone growth result in limb shortening and bowing deformities of the distal limbs; afebrile; nonpainful; heritable

CBC/BIOCHEMISTRY/URINALYSIS
- Do not contribute to diagnosis
- Stress leukogram
- Normal serum parameters
- Hypocalcemia uncommon

OTHER LABORATORY TESTS
N/A

IMAGING
- Distal extremity radiographs—irregular radiolucent zones within metaphyses, parallel and adjacent to physes; flared metaphyses; extraperiosteal new bone extending up the diaphyses; mineralization of perimetaphyseal soft

tissues; asynchronous growth in paired bones; cranial bowing; valgus deformity
- Vertebrae and mandible—rarely affected
- Thoracic radiographs—may reveal interstitial infiltrates

DIAGNOSTIC PROCEDURES
N/A

PATHOLOGIC FINDINGS
- Distal metaphyses of the radius and ulna—most severe changes; similar abnormalities in all long bones
- Gross—wide metaphyses; peripheral mineralization; soft tissue swelling

Histologic
- Nonseptic suppurative inflammation of the metaphysis (osteochondritis), especially adjacent to growth plates
- Necrosis and probable secondary failure of osseous tissue deposition onto the calcified cartilage lattice of the primary spongiosa
- Trabecular microfractures and impaction
- Defective bone formation—thought to be secondary to osteochondral complex inflammation
- Mineralization of perimetaphyseal soft tissues and soft tissues in other regions of the body
- Interstitial pneumonia

 TREATMENT

APPROPRIATE HEALTH CARE
- None specific
- Supportive—from none to intensive care for severely affected puppies
- Depends on the severity of the episode, pyrexia, and the patient's ability to maintain normal hydration and willingness to eat

NURSING CARE
- Some patients will not stand or move—prone to develop pressure sores; turn every 2–4 hr to prevent sores and hypostatic congestion of the dependent lung
- Intravenous fluid therapy—for dehydration; maintenance fluid thereafter

HYPERTROPHIC OSTEODYSTROPHY

ACTIVITY
- Restricted—running and jumping may exacerbate metaphyseal injury and result in further inflammation.
- Confine to a small well-padded area—recommended
- Leash walking only

DIET
- Normal commercial puppy ration
- Avoid supplements

CLIENT EDUCATION
- Warn the client of the disease's relapsing nature.
- Inform client that bony deformities will remodel to some degree with time but that bowing and valgus deformations are permanent.
- Warn client that the more severe the disease, the more severe the bowing deformity.

SURGICAL CONSIDERATIONS
- Generally none
- Consider surgical methods of alimentation (pharyngostomy tube, esophagostomy tube, gastrostomy tube)—debilitated puppies that will not eat or drink and have frequently relapsing episodes of acute clinical signs

 MEDICATIONS

DRUG(S) OF CHOICE
- Antiinflammatory drugs—for pain and antipyretic effects; may try aspirin (10 mg/kg PO q12h), carprofen (1–2 mg/kg IM or PO q12h), or etodalac (10–15 mg/kg PO q24h)
- Prednisone—0.5–1.0 mg/kg PO q24h); only when there is no response to NSAIDs

CONTRAINDICATIONS
Vitamin C—may be contraindicated; may accelerate dystrophic calcification and decrease bone remodeling

PRECAUTIONS
- Avoid immunosuppressive drugs if an infectious cause is proven or if secondary infection is seen.
- NSAIDs—may cause gastric ulceration; watch for hematemesis or melena.

POSSIBLE INTERACTIONS
None

ALTERNATIVE DRUG(S)
None

 FOLLOW-UP

PATIENT MONITORING
Signs of improvement—less metaphyseal sensitivity; patient gets up; appetite improves; pyrexia resolves.

PREVENTION/AVOIDANCE
N/A

POSSIBLE COMPLICATIONS
- Cachexia
- Permanent bowing deformities
- Secondary bacterial infection
- Pressure sores
- Muscle fasciculations, seizure—with hypocalcemia
- May see secondary septicemia

EXPECTED COURSE AND PROGNOSIS
- Course—days to weeks
- Most patients—one or two episodes and recover
- Some patients—seem to have intractable relapsing episodes of pain and pyrexia; rarely die or are euthanized
- Prognosis—usually good; guarded with multiple relapses or complicating secondary problems
- Persistent bowing deformity—eliminates many purebred puppies from the show ring

 MISCELLANEOUS

ASSOCIATED CONDITIONS
Craniomandibular osteopathy—may be associated with mineralization of soft tissues (ossifying periostitis) around long bones; similar to hypertrophic osteodystrophy; may result in lameness

HYPERTROPHIC OSTEODYSTROPHY

AGE-RELATED FACTORS
None

ZOONOTIC POTENTIAL
None

PREGNANCY
Occurs only in juveniles

SYNONYMS
Metaphyseal osteopathy

SEE ALSO
- Elbow Dysplasia
- Osteochondrosis
- Panosteitis

Suggested Reading

Abeles V, Harrus S, Amgles JM. Hypertrophic osteodystrophy in six Weimaraner puppies associated with systemic signs. Vet Rec 1999;145(5):130–134.

Bellah JR. Hypertrophic osteodystrophy. In: Bojrab MJ, ed. Disease mechanisms in small animal surgery. 2nd ed. Philadelphia: Lea & Febiger, 1993:858–864.

Lenehan TM, Fetter AW. Hypertrophic osteodystrophy. In: Newton CD, Nunamaker DM, eds. Textbook of small animal orthopedics. Philadelphia: Lippincott, 1985:597–601.

Mee AP, Gordon MT, May C, et al. Canine virus transcripts detected in the bone cells of dogs with metaphyseal osteopathy. Bone 1993;14:59–67.

Schulz KS, Payne JT, Aronson E. Escherichia coli bacteremia associated with hypertrophic osteodystrophy in a dog. JAVMA 1991;199:1170–1173.

Author: Jamie R. Bellah
Consulting Editor: Peter K. Shires

Hypertrophic Osteopathy

 BASICS

OVERVIEW
- Results in increased peripheral blood flow and periosteal new bone proliferation along the diaphyseal region of long bones, often beginning in the distal phalanges, metacarpals, and metatarsals
- Pathogenesis—speculative; theories: chronic anoxia, obscure toxins, hyperestrogenism, and autonomic neurovascular reflex mechanisms mediated by afferent branches of the vagus or intercostal nerves
- Considered a manifestation of a primary disease process
- Affects the musculoskeletal system

SIGNALMENT
- More common in dogs than cats
- Age of highest frequency—8 years; coincides with the peak incidence of pulmonary neoplasms
- Mean age—5.6 years for dogs with nonneoplastic lung lesions
- Large-breed dogs—12 years of age with embryonal rhabdomyosarcoma

SIGNS

Historical Findings
- Listlessness
- Reluctance to move
- Enlargement of the distal portion of the extremities

Physical Examination Findings
- Lame, sore, and painful limbs
- Extremities—enlarged and firm to the touch; not edematous
- Swelling—predominantly below level of elbow and stifle joints, extending distally to toes

HYPERTROPHIC OSTEOPATHY

CAUSES & RISK FACTORS
- Primary and metastatic lung tumors
- Nonneoplastic thoracic conditions—pneumonia; heartworm disease; congenital or acquired heart disease; bronchial foreign bodies; *Spirocerca lupi* infestation of esophagus; focal lung atelectasis
- Esophageal sarcoma
- Embryonal rhabdomyosarcoma of the urinary bladder
- Adenocarcinoma of the liver or prostate gland
- Thoracic and abdominal mesotheliomas

 DIAGNOSIS

DIFFERENTIAL DIAGNOSIS
- Osteomyelitis—not symmetrical and generally edematous; lysis; history of penetrating trauma or systemic infection
- Metastatic neoplasia—not symmetrical

CBC/BIOCHEMISTRY/URINALYSIS
- Depend on the underlying cause
- Serum ALP—may be elevated

OTHER LABORATORY TESTS
Ultrasound—help identify and differentiate primary lesions

IMAGING
- Radiographs of affected long bones—bilaterally symmetric extensive, rough, periosteal new bone formation on diaphyseal regions; buds project outward from the cortex and perpendicular to the long axis; periosteal new bone forms around the entire circumference of the bone; joints not affected
- Radiographs of the thoracic and abdominal cavities—indicated; identify underlying cause

DIAGNOSTIC PROCEDURES
Bone biopsy and culture (bacterial and fungal)—necessary only in atypical cases; rule out neoplasia and osteomyelitis

TREATMENT

- Directed at underlying primary cause
- Options in selected cases—unilateral vagotomy on the side of a lung lesion; incising through parietal pleura; subperiosteal rib resection; bilateral cervical vagotomy

MEDICATIONS

DRUG(S)
- Depend on underlying cause
- Glucocorticoids (e.g., prednisone)—may be used to improve clinical signs and reduce the extent of swelling
- Analgesics—as needed

CONTRAINDICATIONS/POSSIBLE INTERACTIONS
N/A

FOLLOW-UP

PATIENT MONITORING
- Condition indicates other disease processes—important to recognize need for further diagnostic tests to identify the primary cause
- Removal of the inciting cause—may bring about regression of clinical signs

EXPECTED COURSE AND PROGNOSIS
- Bony changes—may take several months to regress
- Prognosis—guarded to poor owing to the common occurrence of neoplastic causes

MISCELLANEOUS

SYNONYMS
- Hypertrophic pulmonary osteopathy (HPO)
- Hypertrophic pulmonary osteoarthropathy (HPOA)
- Hypertrophic osteoarthropathy (HOA)

HYPERTROPHIC OSTEOPATHY

ABBREVIATION
ALP = alkaline phosphatase

Suggested Reading
Halliwell WH. Tumorlike lesions of bone. In: Bojrab MJ, ed.
    Disease mechanisms in small animal surgery.
    Philadelphia: Lea & Febiger, 1993:933–934.

Author: Peter D. Schwarz
Consulting Editor: Peter K. Shires

Intervertebral Disc Disease, Cervical

 BASICS

DEFINITION
A degeneration of the cervical intervertebral discs that caus-es protrusion or extrusion of disc material into the spinal canal. The protruded or extruded disc material causes spinal cord compression (myelopathy) and/or nerve root entrap-ment (radiculopathy).

PATHOPHYSIOLOGY
- Classified as acute disc herniation (Hansen type I disc) or chronic disc protrusion (Hansen type II disc).
- Hansen type I disc degeneration is characterized by chon-droid degeneration of the nucleus pulposus and acute rupture of the anulus fibrosus with extrusion of the nucleus pulposus into the spinal canal.
- Hansen type II disc degeneration is characterized by fibri-noid degeneration of the nucleus pulposus. This causes bulging and protrusion of the dorsal anulus fibrosus into the vertebral canal.
- Disc extrusion or protrusion into the spinal canal causes focal compression of the spinal cord (myelopathy) and/or focal compression of a nerve root (radiculopathy).
- Consequences of spinal cord compression are ischemia and demyelination.
- Dorsal disc extrusion or protrusion is more common than lateral disc extrusion or protrusion.
- Disc extrusion may be secondary to trauma.
- Surgical fusion of cervical vertebrae may alter the biome-chanics on adjacent vertebral bodies and therefore pre-dispose discs to protrusion or extrusion.

SYSTEM AFFECTED
- Nervous system—either focal myelopathy or focal radicu-lopathy

INTERVERTEBRAL DISC DISEASE, CERVICAL

GENETICS
- Not known
- Chondrodystrophoid breeds (e.g., dachshunds, beagles, cocker spaniels) are most commonly affected with Hansen type I disc extrusion.
- Large breed dogs (e.g., Doberman pinschers) are most commonly affected with Hansen type II disc extrusion.

INCIDENCE/PREVALENCE
- Cervical disc disease accounts for roughly 15% of all canine intervertebral disc disease.
- Eighty percent of disc extrusion occurs in dachshunds, beagles, and poodles.
- C3–C4 is reported to be the most common site of disc extrusion.

SIGNALMENT

Species
Dogs

Breed Predisposition
- Hansen type I—dachshunds, poodles, beagles, cocker spaniels
- Hansen type II—Doberman pinschers

Mean Age and Range
- Hansen type I—3–6 years of age
- Hansen type II—8–10 years of age

Predominant Sex
None recognized

SIGNS
Severity of clinical signs and spinal cord injury is dependent on several factors, including the rate and volume of disc extrusion or protrusion, spinal cord diameter relative to vertebral canal diameter, and the velocity of disc material that was extruded.

Historical Findings
- Neck pain—most common owner complaint
- Stiff, stilted gait, reluctance to move the head and neck
- Lowered head stance and muscle spasms of the head and neck

- It has been reported that 10% of affected patients are tetraparetic.
- Muscle atrophy over the scapula
- Patients may have neck pain and front leg lameness secondary to dorsolateral disc extrusion.

Physical Examination Findings

- Neck pain—elicited upon flexion and extension of the neck or by turning the neck from side to side. Pain can also be elicited by deep palpation of the cervical muscles.
- Occasionally patients have neck pain and apparent forelimb lameness as a result of dorsolateral disc herniation (root signature/radiculopathy). This helps localize the lesion to C4–C7.
- Paresis with postural reaction deficits involving both thoracic and pelvic limbs may be present. The deficits can also be ipsilateral in nature.
- Pelvic limb paresis may be more severe than thoracic limb paresis.
- Pelvic limb spinal reflexes may be normal to exaggerated.
- Thoracic limb spinal reflexes may be normal to exaggerated when lesions are located in the C1–C6 spinal cord segments and may be normal to decreased when the C6–T2 spinal cord segment is affected.
- Bladder function may be upper motor neuron in nature or normal.

CAUSES

- Hansen type I—early chondroid degeneration of the cervical intervertebral disc and subsequent disc mineralization
- Hansen type II—gradual fibroid degeneration of the cervical intervertebral disc

RISK FACTORS

Obesity and repeated traumatic events

 DIAGNOSIS

DIFFERENTIAL DIAGNOSIS

- Hansen type I disc disease
- Hansen type II disc disease

INTERVERTEBRAL DISC DISEASE, CERVICAL

- Neoplasia
- Atlantoaxial instability
- Discospondylitis
- Meningitis
- Fibrocartilaginous embolism
- Cervical vertebral instability
- Spinal fracture/luxation
- Endocrine—hypothyroidism

CBC/BIOCHEMISTRY/URINALYSIS
Should be performed in older animals in anticipation of general anesthesia and surgery

OTHER LABORATORY TESTS
- Cerebrospinal fluid (CSF) analysis—performed under general anesthesia prior to myelography. CSF should be collected from a cisternal tap since this site is closer to the lesion than a lumbar tap.
- CSF analysis reveals mild to moderate elevation in protein levels and mild to moderate pleocytosis.
- Hansen type I disc herniation is usually associated with more severe CSF changes than in Hansen type II disc disease.

IMAGING

Cervical Spinal Radiography
- Well-positioned lateral and ventrodorsal survey radiographs of the cervical spine are always indicated.
- Animals should be anesthetized for this procedure.
- Classic findings include narrowed intervertebral disc space, collapse of the articular facets, calcified disc material present in the intervertebral foramen or in the spinal canal
- Hansen type II disc disease may be associated with spondylosis deformans.
- May reveal evidence of discospondylitis, fracture/luxation, atlantoaxial instability, or lytic vertebrae suggestive of a bone tumor

Myelography
- Myelography is indicated in 90% to 95% of cervical disc patients.

- Survey cervical radiographs may be misleading.
- Either a cisternal or lumbar injection between L5 and L6 or L4 and L5 can be used.
- Lateral radiographs—reveal dorsal deviation of the ventral contrast column over the intervertebral disc space consistent with an extradural mass
- An intraforaminal or dorsolateral disc herniation is best seen on an oblique cervical radiograph, with the entire cervical spine positioned at a 45- to 60-degree angle to the table.

Enhanced Diagnostic Imaging
Magnetic resonance imaging (MRI) and computed tomography have also been used for diagnosis of cervical intervertebral disc disease.

DIAGNOSTIC PROCEDURES
Cerebral spinal fluid analysis

PATHOLOGIC FINDINGS

Gross Findings
- Hansen type I disc—white extruded disc material that has a granular consistency and is usually easily removed from the spinal canal
- Hansen type II disc—firm protrusion of the dorsal annulus fibrosus that is adherent to the floor of the spinal canal and to the dura of the spinal cord. Type II discs are much more difficult to remove from the spinal canal.
- Spinal cord—in acute disc extrusion the spinal cord may appear bruised and swollen; in chronic disc protrusion the spinal cord may appear to be atrophied but is often normal in appearance.

Histopathologic Findings
- Hansen type I disc—shifting concentration of glycosaminoglycans, loss of water and proteoglycan content, and increased collagen content. The disc becomes more cartilaginous and undergoes dystrophic calcification.
- Hansen type II disc—a gradual fibroid metaplasia leaves the disc with increased glycosaminoglycan level and lower collagen content. The nucleus does not undergo cartilaginous metaplasia.

INTERVERTEBRAL DISC DISEASE, CERVICAL

- Spinal cord—dependent on the severity of the disease and type of disc disease. Hansen type II—demyelination and gliosis are seen. Hansen type I—hemorrhage and edema can be seen and with severe disease myelomalacia can be observed

 TREATMENT

APPROPRIATE HEALTH CARE
- Conservative management—dependent on patient's history and presenting neurologic status
- Surgical management—patients with repeated episodes of neck pain, patients presented with severe neck pain and neurologic deficits, or patients that have not responded to conservative management

NURSING CARE
- Handling—minimal manipulation of the cervical spine and avoidance of jugular venipuncture if at all possible
- Urination—monitor patients for complete emptying of the bladder; patients may need to have bladder manually expressed or intermittent bladder catheterization. In some cases indwelling urinary catheter may need to be placed. Urinalysis, including culture and sensitivity, should be performed after removal of an indwelling catheter to make sure the patient did not obtain a nosocomial bacterial cystitis.
- Defecation—patients may need enemas and can be switched to a low-residue diet to decrease the volume of feces
- Recumbent patients—should be kept on a well-padded mat and turned every 4 hours. Patients should be checked for pressure sores over bony prominences, which can lead to prolonged hospital stays and more surgeries.
- Physical therapy—hydrotherapy and passive range of motion of all joints should be performed as often as possible to prevent severe muscle atrophy

ACTIVITY
- Minimal, no running or jumping. When patients are being leash-walked, a harness should be used instead of a collar.

- With conservative management patients should be strictly confined to cage rest for 3 to 4 weeks.
- Following surgery patients should have minimal activity and be leash-walked only for 4 to 6 weeks, then slowly re-introduced to full activity.

DIET
For obese patients, a reducing diet should be instituted.

CLIENT EDUCATION
- For conservative management, strict cage confinement should be emphasized.
- Weight loss if the animal is obese
- Common clinical signs of animals with cervical disc disease

SURGICAL CONSIDERATIONS
- When indicated the goal of surgery is to remove disc material from the spinal canal and therefore decompress the spinal cord and/or nerve root.
- Surgery usually provides immediate pain relief and eventual normal motor function.
- A ventral cervical slot is the most common surgical approach for the removal of disc material from the spinal canal.
- Disc material that has extruded dorsolaterally into the intervertebral foramen is removed via a lateral approach to the cervical spine or through a dorsal laminectomy, with or without a facetectomy.
- Fenestration alone for dogs with neck pain only usually does not resolve clinical signs.

 MEDICATIONS

DRUG(S)
- Low-dose glucocorticoid therapy may be beneficial in order to decrease the pain in animals that are being treated conservatively.
- Glucocorticoids given to animals without simultaneous strict cage confinement could exacerbate disc extrusion by encouraging exercise.

INTERVERTEBRAL DISC DISEASE, CERVICAL

- Methylprednisolone sodium succinate—30 mg/kg intravenously within the first 8 hr of clinical onset can be given in acute cases. This can be followed by a dose of 15 mg/kg 2 hr after the initial dose, then every 6 hr for 24 hr.
- If high-dose steroid therapy is initiated, gastrointestinal protectants should also be given. Common drugs used are cimetidine, ranitidine, misoprostol, and sucralfate.
- Nonsteroidal antiinflammatory drugs (NSAIDs) should be avoided, since they may cause severe gastric irritation and ulceration.
- Muscle relaxants can be used, but are generally unsuccessful when used alone.

CONTRAINDICATIONS
Never use glucocorticoids simultaneously with NSAIDs—this can cause severe gastrointestinal irritation and possibly intestinal perforation.

PRECAUTIONS
When using high-dose corticosteroids for cervical disc disease, patients should be placed on gastro-protectants to prevent the gastrointestinal side effects associated with corticosteroids.

POSSIBLE INTERACTIONS
NSAIDs in combination with glucocorticoids can cause gastrointestinal perforation or severe gastrointestinal bleeding, both situations leading to death.

 FOLLOW-UP

PATIENT MONITORING
- Weekly evaluations should be performed until the resolution of clinical signs.
- All patients should be fitted with a harness, and neck collars should be avoided.

PREVENTION/AVOIDANCE
- Inherent in particular breeds
- Keeping patients at an ideal weight may help.

POSSIBLE COMPLICATIONS
- Complications are uncommon.
- Continued neck pain
- Deteriorating motor status
- Subluxation/luxation of vertebral bodies

EXPECTED COURSE AND PROGNOSIS
- Prognosis for patients treated surgically or conservatively depends on neurologic signs at the time of presentation.
- Prognosis is generally favorable for most patients.
- Most patients treated conservatively have recurrence of disease and may require surgical intervention.

 MISCELLANEOUS

ASSOCIATED CONDITIONS
Animals predisposed to cervical disc disease are also the same breeds that are predisposed to thoracolumbar disc disease.

SEE ALSO
Intervertebral Disc Disease, Thoracolumbar

Suggested Reading
Oliver JE, Lorenz MD, Kornegay JN. Handbook of veterinary neurology. 3rd ed. Philadelphia: Saunders, 1997: 174–187.
Seim HB. Surgery of the cervical spine. In: Small animal surgery. 2nd ed. St. Louis: Mosby, 2002:1213–1268.
Toombs JP: Cervical intervertebral disc disease in dogs. Compend Contin Educ Pract Vet 1992;14:1477.

Acknowledgment
The author and editors acknowledge the prior contributions of Mary O. Smith, who authored this topic in the previous edition.

Author: Otto L. Lanz
Consulting Editor: Peter K. Shires

Intervertebral Disc Disease, Thoracolumbar

 BASICS

DEFINITION
Degenerative changes within the intervertebral discs characterized by loss of water, cellular necrosis, and calcification. Biomechanical properties of the disc deteriorate, resulting in extrusion or protrusion of disc material.

PATHOPHYSIOLOGY
- Accelerated degeneration of discs in chondrodystrophic breeds has been termed chondroid metaplasia.
- Hansen Type I refers to acute extrusion of nucleus pulposus through the annulus into the vertebral canal; typically occurs in small chondrodystrophic breeds but may occur in larger non-chondrodystrophic dogs as well.
- Hansen Type II lesions involve gradual protrusion (bulging) of the dorsal anular fibers into the vertebral canal; this is associated with fibroid metaplasia of the disc.
- Acute disc extrusion results in disc material causing direct spinal cord injury and disc mass causing spinal cord compression. Disc mass (spinal cord compression) results in ischemia and spinal cord changes that vary from mild demyelination to necrosis of both gray and white matter; events at the cellular level include release of vasoactive substances, increased intracellular calcium, and increased free radical formation and lipid peroxides.
- Pain due to dural irritation, nerve root impingement, or possibly discogenic in origin
- Disc herniation rare between T3 and T10 owing to presence of intercapital ligament

SYSTEM AFFECTED
Nervous

INTERVERTEBRAL DISC DISEASE, THORACOLUMBAR

GENETICS
Chondrodystrophic breeds (e.g., dachshunds, shih tzu, Pekingese) are predisposed to Hansen type I disease; larger breeds more commonly have Hansen type II disease.

INCIDENCE/PREVALENCE
- Most common neurologic dysfunction in small animals; affects 2% of the canine population
- Rarely occurs in felines
- Thoracolumbar disc disease comprises 85% of all disc herniations.

SIGNALMENT

Species
Dogs and occasionally cats

Breed Predilections
- Type I—Dachshunds, shih tzus, Lhaso apso, Pekingese, cocker spaniels, Welsh corgis, toy and miniature poodles
- Type II—large breeds but may occur in any breed

Mean Age and Range
- Type I—3–7 years of age
- Type II—8–10 years of age; cats mean age of 10 years

SIGNS

General Comments
Signs depend on the type of herniation, the velocity of disc contact with the spinal cord, the amount and duration of cord compression, the location (UMN or LMN), and the spinal canal/spinal cord diameter ratio (cervical vs. thoracolumbar).

Historical Findings
- Onset may be peracute or acute in chondrodystrophoid dogs (type I disease), and may occur during vigorous activity.
- Larger dogs or smaller dogs with type II disease have a more insidious onset, and tend to worsen with time.

INTERVERTEBRAL DISC DISEASE, THORACOLUMBAR

Physical Examination Findings

- Varies considerably depending on type of herniation and anatomic location of lesion
- Thoracolumbar pain common in dogs; reluctant to ambulate and hunched posture; careful palpation of spinous processes and epaxial musculature produces distinct localized pain; often some degree of paraparesis with decreased or absent proprioception in the rear limbs
- Spinal reflexes in the rear limbs are usually exaggerated (hyper) when lesion is between T3 and L3; reflexes are decreased (hypo) when lesion is caudal to L3.
- 75% of thoracolumbar herniations occur between T11 and L3.
- Superficial and deep pain perception may be decreased or absent in the rear limbs; presence of deep pain sensation is the single most reliable prognostic factor for return to acceptable function; pain perception should be cerebral in nature and not confused with a withdrawal reflex (local spinal reflex).
- Forelimb function is normal; occasionally Schiff-Sherrington phenomena may cause increased muscle tone in the forelimbs.
- Urinary incontinence or retention is common when the lesion affects motor function.
- Pain is less obvious in cats; the site of herniation is often lumbar.

CAUSES

- Chondroid or fibroid degeneration of the thoracolumbar intervertebral discs
- 15% of animals with spinal fractures have been reported to have disc extrusions in addition to the fracture/luxation.

RISK FACTORS

Type I disease most often affects chondrodystrophic breeds.

DIAGNOSIS

DIFFERENTIAL DIAGNOSIS
- Type I—Trauma causing fracture/luxation, neoplasia, discospondylitis, fibrocartilaginous embolism; differentiated by history, survey radiography, and myelography
- Type II—degenerative myelopathy, neoplasia, discospondylitis, orthopedic disease; differentiated by history, radiography, and careful orthopedic and neurologic examination

CBC/BIOCHEMISTRY/URINALYSIS
- Elevation of liver enzymes common if patient has received corticosteroids for pain or neurologic disease
- Urine retention/incontinence increases risk of urinary tract infection characterized by leukocytes, protein, and bacteruria on urinalysis.

OTHER LABORATORY TESTS
CSF analysis performed routinely in conjunction with myelography and if there is high suspicion of another disease process; may be normal but more typically shows mild to moderate increase in protein with or without pleocytosis

IMAGING
- Thoracolumbar spinal radiography
- Survey radiographs rule out some other disease processes.
- Diagnostic radiographs taken under general anesthesia may reveal a narrowed or wedged disc space, collapsed articular facet space, and small intervertebral foramen with increased or mineralized density within the spinal canal.

DIAGNOSTIC PROCEDURES
- Myelography performed with iohexol recommended in all patients when surgery is indicated; contrast usually introduced at L5–L6; usually shows an extradural mass lesion causing spinal cord compression adjacent to the affected disc; spinal cord swelling may be evidenced by

thinning of contrast columns over several intervertebral spaces
- CT, MRI, or repeat myelography may be indicated when results are not definitive.
- CSF analysis

PATHOLOGIC FINDINGS

Gross
- Extruded disc material (type I disease)—white to yellow and "toothpaste" consistency; if chronic, may be hardened and adhered to surrounding structures.
- Protruded disc material (type II disease)—usually firm, grayish white and may be adherent to surrounding structures
- Spinal cord may appear normal or be swollen and discolored in acute severe disease.

Histopathologic
- Degenerated discs have decreased amounts of proteoglycans, glycosaminoglycans, and water; discs may become mineralized or cartilaginous.
- Spinal cord lesion depends upon type and severity of disc extrusion or protrusion; acute, severe disease may cause hemorrhage, edema, tissue necrosis; chronic disease demyelination of white and in some cases gray matter

 TREATMENT

APPROPRIATE HEALTH CARE
- Guidelines for therapy based on classification of clinical condition
  Class 1—back-pain only
  Class 2—back pain, ataxia, mild paraparesis, motor ability good
  Class 3—proprioceptive deficits, motor ability affected but still present
  Class 4—complete paraparesis (no motor ability) with deep pain perception present
  Class 5—complete paraparesis, no deep pain present
- Class 1 patients treated medically

- Class 2 patients treated medically initially with serial neurologic exam, surgery if patient remains static or condition declines
- Classes 3 and 4 surgical therapy
- Class 5 surgical therapy if within the first 12–24 hours of occurrence
- Serial neurologic examination important for all affected animals

NURSING CARE

- Absolute restricted confinement for 2–4 weeks
- Minimize spinal manipulation and support spine when handling patient.
- Ensure ability to urinate or consider bladder expression, intermittent catheterization, or indwelling urinary catheter for patients in classes 3–5
- Recumbent patients should be kept clean on padded bedding placed on elevated cage racks and turned frequently to prevent formation of decubital ulcers.
- Manual evacuation of the bowel or enemas may be necessary to promote defecation.
- Physical therapy with passive manipulation of rear limbs begun early followed by more intense therapy (hydrotherapy) for animals with neurologic deficits
- Carts useful in many patients in promoting return to function; patient tolerance is limiting factor.

ACTIVITY

- Restricted movement most important part of medical management
- Cage rest in hospital or enforced cage rest as an outpatient for 2–4 weeks for class 1 patients or postoperative animals

DIET

Weight reduction if patient is obese

CLIENT EDUCATION

- Describe signs of spinal cord compression and advise client of need for reevaluation in the case of worsening clinical signs.

INTERVERTEBRAL DISC DISEASE, THORACOLUMBAR

- Emphasize the importance of restricted activity and how that may be accomplished when treating the patient medically or following surgery.
- Some degree of restricted activity may be important for the remainder of the animals's life since it has disc disease.
- Most animals in classes 1–4 have a good to excellent prognosis for return to function, i.e., ambulation with bowel and bladder continence; patients in class 5 have a poorer but not hopeless prognosis; percentages vary but up to approximately 50% may regain deep pain and some function.

SURGICAL CONSIDERATIONS
- Strongly indicated for animals in classes 3 and 4, also within the first 12–24 hours for class 5 dogs; also indicated for static or worsening class 1 and 2 dogs
- Primary surgical goal is to relieve spinal cord compression by disc mass removal via hemilaminectomy, dorsal laminectomy, or pediculectomy; disk fenestration alone rarely indicated
- Recurrence of clinical signs in animals who have been operated on may be due to further extrusion of disc from the original site in many cases.
- Surgical controversies remain over the issues of prophylactic disc fenestration performed concurrently with decompressive surgery and the prognosis for return to function after surgery in negative deep pain patients.

 MEDICATIONS

DRUG(S) OF CHOICE
- Methylprednisolone sodium succinate—30 mg/kg IV, within 8 hours of onset or presurgically in classes 2–5; some clinicians recommend repeat administration 12 hours later of 30 mg/kg or at 15 mg/kg 2 and 6 hours after first dose for severe acute disease (classes 4 and 5)
- Prednisone or prednisolone—0.25–0.50 mg/kg PO twice daily for 2–4 days, then taper dose over 10 days for

animals not having surgery; important that therapy be combined with strict cage rest and repeated neurologic examinations
- NSAIDs may be used as an analgesic in class 1 cases rather than prednisone or prednisolone.
- Narcotic analgesics may be necessary postoperatively; oxymorphone (0.05–0.1 mg/kg IV or IM q4h), butorphanol (0.2–0.4 mg/kg IV, IM, or SC every 2–4 hours), or buprenorphine (5–15 μg/kg IV or IM q6h)
- Methocarbamol (25–45 mg/kg q8h) may be useful in cases where muscle spasm is contributing to pain; more applicable with cervical disease
- Bethanechol (5–15 mg/dog PO) and phenoxybenzamine (0.25 mg/kg PO q8–12h) variably helpful in managing bladder dysfunction associated with spinal cord lesion.

CONTRAINDICATIONS
Avoid concomitant use of glucocorticoids and NSAIDs because of combined negative effects on the gastrointestinal tract.

PRECAUTIONS
- Use of glucocorticoids without cage confinement may decrease pain, thereby encouraging excessive activity and leading to further disc herniation and deterioration of clinical condition.
- High doses of glucocorticoids such as dexamethasone especially in combination with surgical therapy may result in extensive gastrointestinal hemorrhage and intestinal perforation; less common with other glucocorticoids

ALTERNATIVE DRUG(S) & THERAPIES
- Acupuncture may be effective for animals with chronic pain where no compressive lesion can be demonstrated by myelography.
- Discolysis by enzymatic injection or laser ablation described but not proven therapy in dogs

FOLLOW-UP

PATIENT MONITORING
- Patients treated medically should be re-evaluated 2–3 times daily for worsening neurologic signs for the first 48 hours after onset
- If stable, re-evaluate daily, then weekly, until clinical signs have resolved.
- Patients treated surgically are evaluated twice daily until improvement is noted; urinary bladder function or awaiting development of an autonomic bladder are the limiting factors for hospitalization.

PREVENTION/AVOIDANCE
Prevention of obesity and avoiding strenuous exercise or jumping may or may not avoid exacerbation of clinical signs.

POSSIBLE COMPLICATIONS
- Recurrence of signs associated with disc herniation at original or at new site
- Deterioration of clinical signs with or without surgery; hard-to-predict clinical course in some cases, especially those with severe type 1 lesions
- Rarely, development of ascending or descending myelomalacia; occurs in class 4 or 5 dogs 3–5 days following injury and characterized by variable and changing neurologic findings, possible fever, possible dyspnea; euthanasia event when diagnosed

EXPECTED COURSE AND PROGNOSIS
- Overall prognosis for dogs in class 1–4 good; those treated conservatively may experience recurrence of clinical signs.
- Recurrence rates of dogs without fenestration at the time of laminectomy range from 5–30%.
- Dogs in class 5 have a variable (10–75%) chance of recovery; overall a guarded prognosis

MISCELLANEOUS

ASSOCIATED CONDITIONS
Predisposed patients and breeds may have concurrent cervical disk disease

SEE ALSO
Intervertebral Disc Disease, Cervical

ABBREVIATIONS
- CSF = cerebrospinal fluid
- NSAID = nonsteroidal antiinflammatory drug

Suggested Reading

Fingeroth JM. Treatment of canine intervertebral disk disease: recommendations and controversies. In Bonagura JD, ed. Current veterinary therapy XII. Philadelphia: Saunders, 1995:1146–1152.

Munana KR, Olby N, Sharp NJH, et al. Intervertebral disc disease in 10 cats. J Am Anim Hosp Assoc 2001;37: 384–389.

Seim HB. Conditions of the thoracolumbar spine. Semin Vet Med Surg 1996; 11:235–253.

Seim HB. Surgery of the thoracolumbar spine. In: Fossum TW, ed. Small Animal Surgery, 2nd ed. St. Louis: Mosby, 2002: 1269–1287.

Acknowledgment

The author/editors acknowledge the prior contributions of Dr. Mary Smith, who authored this topic in the previous edition.

Author: Don R. Waldron
Consulting Editor: Peter K. Shires

Lameness

 BASICS

DEFINITION
A disturbance in gait and locomotion in response to pain or injury

PATHOPHYSIOLOGY
- Severe, sharp pain—when moving, patient carries or puts no weight on the affected limb.
- Milder, dull, or aching pain—when moving, patient limps or bears little weight on the affected limb; at rest, the patient bears less weight on the affected limb.
- Pain produced only during certain phases of movement—patient adjusts its motion and gait to minimize discomfort.

SYSTEMS AFFECTED
- Musculoskeletal
- Nervous

SIGNALMENT
- Any age or breed of dog
- Age, breed, and sex predilection—depend on specific disease

SIGNS

General Comments
- Unilateral forelimb—compensated for by moving the head and neck upward as the affected limb is placed on the ground and dropping the head and neck when the sound limb bears the weight
- Bilateral hindlimb—head and neck movement less pronounced; more weight shifted to the forelimbs by dropping the forequarters
- Unilateral hindlimb—may drop lower on the sound limb when it strikes the ground; elevated hindquarters when the affected limb is on the ground

- Always assess the patient's neurologic status, especially with a suspected proximal lesion.

Historical Findings
- Complete history—mandatory; signalment; identification of affected limb(s); known trauma; changes with weather, exercise, or rest; responsiveness to previous treatments
- Determine onset of lameness—acute or chronic
- Determine progression—static; slow; rapid
- Is the patient demonstrably painful?

Physical Examination Findings
- Perform a complete routine examination.
- Observe gait—walking; trotting; climbing stairs; doing figure-eights
- Palpate—asymmetry of muscle mass; bony prominences
- Manipulate bones and joints, beginning distally and working proximally.
- Assess—instability; incongruency; luxation or subluxation; pain; abnormal range of motion; abnormal sounds
- Examine suspected area of involvement last—by starting with normal limbs, patient may relax, allowing assessment of normal reaction to maneuvers.

CAUSES

Forelimb

Growing Dog (< 12 Months of Age)
- Osteochondrosis of the shoulder
- Shoulder luxation or subluxation—congenital
- Osteochondrosis of the elbow
- Un-united anconeal process
- Fragmented medial coronoid process
- Elbow incongruity
- Avulsion or calcification of the flexor muscles—elbow
- Asymmetric growth of the radius and ulna
- Panosteitis
- Hypertrophic osteodystrophy
- Trauma—soft tissue; bone; joint
- Infection—local; systemic
- Nutritional imbalances
- Congenital anomalies

LAMENESS

Mature Dog (> 12 Months of Age)

- Degenerative joint disease
- Bicipital tenosynovitis
- Calcification or mineralization of supraspinatus or infraspinatus tendon
- Contracture of supraspinatus or infraspinatus muscle
- Soft tissue or bone neoplasia—primary; metastatic
- Trauma—soft tissue; bone; joint
- Panosteitis
- Polyarthropathies
- Polymyositis
- Polyneuritis

Hindlimb

Growing Dog (< 12 Months of Age)

- Hip dysplasia
- Avascular necrosis of femoral head—Legg-Calvé-Perthes disease
- Osteochondrosis of stifle
- Patella luxation—medial or lateral condyle
- Osteochondrosis of hock
- Panosteitis
- Hypertrophic osteodystrophy
- Trauma—soft tissue; bone; joint
- Infection—local; systemic
- Nutritional imbalances
- Congenital anomalies

Mature Dog (> 12 Months of age)

- Degenerative joint disease
- Cruciate ligament disease
- Avulsion of long digital extensor tendon—stifle
- Soft tissue or bone neoplasia—primary; metastatic
- Trauma—soft tissue; bone; joint
- Panosteitis
- Polyarthropathies
- Polymyositis
- Polyneuritis

RISK FACTORS
N/A

DIAGNOSIS

DIFFERENTIAL DIAGNOSIS
Must differentiate musculoskeletal from neurogenic causes

CBC/BIOCHEMISTRY/URINALYSIS
Usually normal

OTHER LABORATORY TESTS
Depend on suspected cause

IMAGING
- Radiographs—recommended for all suspected musculoskeletal causes
- CT, MRI, and bone scans with radioisotopes—help identify and delineate causative lesions

DIAGNOSTIC PROCEDURES
- Cytologic examination of joint fluid—identify and differentiate intraarticular disease
- EMG—differentiate neuromuscular from musculoskeletal disease
- Muscle and/or nerve biopsy—reveal and identify neuromuscular disease

 TREATMENT

Depends on underlying cause

 MEDICATIONS

DRUG(S) OF CHOICE
- Analgesics and NSAIDs—often indicated for symptomatic treatment; try buffered or enteric-coated aspirin (10–25 mg/kg PO q8–12h), carprofen (2.2 mg/kg PO q12h), etodolac (10–15 mg/kg PO q24h), phenylbutazone (3–7 mg/kg PO q8h, total dose < 800 mg/day), meclofenamic acid (0.5 mg/kg PO q12h), or piroxicam (0.3 mg/kg PO q24h for 3 days, then q48h)

LAMENESS

- Corticosteroids—use judiciously, unless specifically indicated (potential side effects; articular cartilage damage associated with long-term use)

CONTRAINDICATIONS
N/A

PRECAUTIONS
NSAIDs—gastrointestinal irritation may preclude use in some patients

POSSIBLE INTERACTIONS
N/A

ALTERNATIVE DRUG(S)
Chondroprotective drugs (e.g., polysulfated glycosaminoglycans, glucosamine, and chondroitin sulfate)—for degenerative joint disease; may be of benefit in limiting cartilage damage and degeneration; may help alleviate pain and inflammation

 FOLLOW-UP

PATIENT MONITORING
Depends on underlying cause

POSSIBLE COMPLICATIONS
N/A

 MISCELLANEOUS

ASSOCIATED CONDITIONS
N/A

AGE-RELATED FACTORS
N/A

ZOONOTIC POTENTIAL
N/A

PREGNANCY
N/A

SEE ALSO
Chapters covering musculoskeletal and neuromuscular disorders

ABBREVIATIONS
- CT = computed tomography
- EMG = electromyogram
- MRI = magnetic resonance imaging
- NSAIDs = nonsteroidal antiinflammatory drugs

Suggested Reading
Brinker WO, Piermattei DL, Flo GL. Physical examination for lameness. In: Handbook of small animal orthopedics and fracture repair. 3rd ed. Philadelphia: Saunders, 1997: 228–230.

Author: Peter D. Schwarz
Consulting Editor: Peter K. Shires

Legg-Calvé-Perthes Disease

 BASICS

DEFINITION
A spontaneous degeneration of the femoral head and neck leading to collapse of the coxofemoral joint and osteoarthritis

PATHOPHYSIOLOGY
- Precise cause unknown; a specific vascular lesion not identified
- Histologic evidence—points to infarction of vessels serving the proximal femur
- Necrosis of subchondral bone—leading to collapse and deformation of the femoral head during normal loading
- Articular cartilage—becomes thickened; cleft development; fraying of superficial layers
- Simultaneous osseous degeneration and repair—characteristic of ischemia and revascularization of bone
- No evidence of hypercoagulability or other blood clotting abnormalities

SYSTEMS AFFECTED
Musculoskeletal—causes a hind leg lameness; insidious in onset

GENETICS
- Manchester terriers—multifactorial inheritance pattern with a high degree of heritability
- Hereditary predisposition likely

INCIDENCE/PREVALENCE
- Common among miniature, toy, and small dog breeds
- No accurate estimates available

GEOGRAPHIC DISTRIBUTION
N/A

SIGNALMENT

Species
Dogs

Breed Predilections
- Toy breeds and terriers—most susceptible
- Manchester terriers, miniature pinschers, toy poodles, Lakeland terriers, west Highland white terriers, and cairn terriers—higher than expected incidence

Mean Age and Range
- Most patients are 5–8 months of age.
- Range—3–13 months

Predominant Sex
None

SIGNS

General Comments
Usually unilateral; only 12%–16% of cases are bilateral.

Historical Findings
Lameness—usually gradual onset over 2–3 months; weight-bearing; occasionally leg is carried.

Physical Examination Findings
- Pain on manipulation of the hip—most common
- Crepitation of the joint—inconsistent
- Atrophy of the thigh muscles—nearly always noted
- Patient otherwise normal

CAUSES
- Unknown
- Tamponade of the intracapsular subsynovial vessels serving the femoral head—suggested cause of ischemia leading to the pathologic changes

RISK FACTORS
- Small, toy, and miniature breeds—increased risk
- Trauma to the hip region

 DIAGNOSIS

DIFFERENTIAL DIAGNOSIS
- Medial patellar luxation—may occur independently; primary differential in young dogs
- Rupture of the cranial cruciate ligament—primary differential in old dogs

LEGG-CALVÉ-PERTHES DISEASE

CBC/BIOCHEMISTRY/URINALYSIS
N/A

OTHER LABORATORY TESTS
N/A

IMAGING
- Early radiographic changes—widening of the joint space; decreased bone density of the epiphysis; sclerosis and thickening of the femoral neck
- Later radiographic changes—lucent areas within the femoral head
- End-stage radiographic changes—flattening and extreme deformation of the femoral head; severe osteoarthrosis

DIAGNOSTIC PROCEDURES
N/A

PATHOLOGIC FINDINGS
- Femoral head—removed during FHNE; usually deformed with a thickened irregular articular surface
- Early disease—histologically characterized by loss of lacunar osteocytes and necrosis of marrow elements; trabeculae surrounded by granulation tissue
- Later disease—thickened metaphyseal trabeculae; mixture of necrosis and repair tissue typical of revascularization of bone
- Advanced disease—osteoclastic activity; new bone formation

 TREATMENT

APPROPRIATE HEALTH CARE
- Rest and analgesics—reportedly successful in alleviating lameness in a minority of patients
- Ehmer sling—successful in one patient; maintained for 10 weeks
- Insidious onset often prevents early recognition and possibility of conservative treatment.
- FHNE with early and vigorous exercise after surgery—treatment of choice

NURSING CARE

Postsurgery
- Physical therapy—extremely important for rehabilitating the affected limb
- Analgesics, anti-inflammatory drugs, and cold packing—3–5 days; important
- Range-of-motion exercises—extension and flexion; initiated immediately
- Small lead weights—attached as ankle bracelets above the hock joint; encourage early use of the treated limb

ACTIVITY
- Postsurgery—early activity encouraged to improve leg use
- Conservative therapy—restricted activity recommended

DIET
Avoid obesity.

CLIENT EDUCATION
- Warn owners of Manchester terriers of the genetic basis of the disease; discourage breeding affected dogs.
- Warn client that recovery after FHNE may take 3–6 months.

SURGICAL CONSIDERATIONS
FHNE—treatment of choice

 MEDICATIONS

DRUG(S) OF CHOICE
NSAIDs—preoperative or postoperatively; minimize joint pain; reduce synovitis; may try buffered or enteric-coated aspirin (10–25 mg/kg PO q8h or q12h), carprofen (2.2 mg/kg PO q12h), etodolac (10–15 mg/kg PO q24h), phenylbutazone (3–7 mg/kg PO q8h, total dose < 800 mg/day), meclofenemic acid (0.5 mg/kg PO q12h), or piroxicam (0.3 mg/kg PO q24h for 3 days, then q48h)

CONTRAINDICATIONS
NSAIDs—gastrointestinal upset may preclude use in some patients.

LEGG-CALVÉ-PERTHES DISEASE

PRECAUTIONS
- NSAIDs—inhibition of platelet activity may increase hemorrhage at surgery; discontinue aspirin for at least 1 week before surgery, if possible; usually cause some degree of gastric ulceration
- Acetaminophen—unsuitable; potential for toxicity

POSSIBLE INTERACTIONS
NSAIDs—do not use in conjunction with glucocorticoids; risk of gastrointestinal tract ulceration

ALTERNATIVE DRUG(S)
Chondroprotective drugs (e.g., polysulfated glycosaminoglycans, glucosamine, and chondroitin sulfate)—little help in advanced disease; no evidence to suggest that these drugs prevent or reverse the disease process

 FOLLOW-UP

PATIENT MONITORING
- Postsurgical progress checks—2-week intervals; necessary to ensure compliance with exercise recommendations
- Conservative therapy—re-evaluated (physical examination, radiographs) to determine if surgery is needed

PREVENTION/AVOIDANCE
- Discourage breeding of affected animals.
- Do not repeat dam–sire breedings that result in affected offspring.

POSSIBLE COMPLICATIONS
Limiting postoperative exercise may result in less than optimal limb function.

EXPECTED COURSE AND PROGNOSIS
- FHNE—good to excellent prognosis for full recovery (84%–100% success rate)
- Conservative therapy—reported to alleviate lameness after 2–3 months in about 25% of patients

MISCELLANEOUS

ASSOCIATED CONDITIONS
N/A

AGE-RELATED FACTORS
Usually affects juvenile small-breed dogs, but maturer dogs may be affected by chronic disease.

ZOONOTIC POTENTIAL
N/A

PREGNANCY
N/A

SYNONYMS
- Perthes disease
- Coxa plana
- Coxa magna
- Avascular necrosis of the femoral head
- Aseptic necrosis of the femoral head
- Osteochondritis juvenilis

SEE ALSO
- Cruciate Disease, Cranial
- Hip Dysplasia—Dogs
- Patella Luxation

ABBREVIATIONS
- FHNE = femoral head and neck excision
- NSAID = nonsteroidal antiinflammatory drug

Suggested Reading
Brenig B, Leeb T, Jansen S, Kopp T. Analysis of blood clotting factor activities in canine Legg-Calvé-Perthes' disease. J Vet Intern Med 1999;13:570–573.

Brinker WO, Piermattei DL, Flo GL, eds. Diagnosis and treatment of orthopedic conditions of the hindlimb. In: Handbook of small animal orthopedics and fracture treatment. 3rd ed. Philadelphia: Saunders 1997:465–466.

Gambardella PC. Legg-Calvé-Perthes disease in dogs. In: Bojrab MJ, ed. Disease mechanisms in small animal surgery. 2nd ed. Philadelphia: Saunders, 1993:804–807.

LEGG-CALVÉ-PERTHES DISEASE

Gibson KL, Lewis DD, Perchman RD. Use of external coaptation for the treatment of avascular necrosis of the femoral head in a dog. J Am Vet Med Assoc 1990; 197:868–869.

Piek, CJ, Hazewinkel HAW, Wolvekamp WTC, et al. Long term follow-up of avascular necrosis of the femoral head in the dog. J Small Anim Pract 1996;37:12–18.

Author: Larry Carpenter
Consulting Editor: Peter K. Shires

Muscle Rupture (Muscle Tear)

 BASICS

OVERVIEW
A normal muscle may be stretched, pinched, or injured directly, resulting in fiber disruption, weakening, and immediate or delayed separation of the uninjured portions. Alternatively the muscle structure may be compromised by systemic or iatrogenic conditions, and normal activity may cause muscle disruption. The rupture may be complete or incomplete, and may be mid-substance or at the muscle-tendon junction. The acute stage is characterized by a typical inflammatory reaction that becomes chronic with collagen maturation, cross-linking, and adhesion development over time. Frequently the acute phase is overlooked as the signs may be temporary and respond well to rest. The chronic effects are often progressive and unresponsive to support therapies.

SIGNALMENT
Limb and masticatory muscles are the primary structures affected. Traumatic injury is indiscriminate, although certain activities may predispose because of exposure. The ruptures that are apparently unrelated to trauma seem to affect middle-aged to older working dogs, with no reported sex predilection. Cats affected less frequently than dogs

SIGNS

Acute Injury
- Immediate lameness that is characterized by the specific muscle affected
- Localized swelling, heat, and pain
- Generally present for a few days to a week

Chronic Phase (if it develops)
- Progressive
- Painless

MUSCLE RUPTURE (MUSCLE TEAR)

- Usually associated with scar tissue that impedes normal function of an extremity

Causes & Risk Factors
- Trauma
- Over-extension
- Myositis
- Degenerative (unknown etiology)
- Myopathy secondary to medical conditions like Cushing's disease
- Apparent risk factor for dogs is involvement in hunting, tracking, or similar activities in the outdoors.

 DIAGNOSIS

DIFFERENTIAL DIAGNOSIS
- Neurologic dysfunction—recognized by neurologic abnormalities
- Tendon rupture—visible or palpable disruption in the tendon
- Origin/insertion avulsion fracture—radiographic evidence of bone fragment defect and translocation
- Luxation/subluxation—palpable or radiographic evidence of joint instability or malalignment

CBC/BIOCHEMISTRY/URINALYSIS
No injury-specific findings

OTHER LABORATORY TESTS
- CPK may be elevated in acute cases.
- No known specific tests available

IMAGING

Radiographic Findings
Soft tissue swelling may be evident in the early stages. Calcification of muscle can occur in the traumatized area in chronic situations.

ULTRASONOGRAPHIC FINDINGS
- Local swelling and disorientation of the normal muscle fiber orientation may be seen at the site of injury in acute cases.

- Scar tissue and contracted areas of fibrous tissue can be seen in the muscle in chronic cases.
- Measurable differences between normal and abnormal sides may be useful in documenting the affected muscle site.

CT Findings
Produces better tissue contrast than the above but still constrained to an axial plane of view.

MRI Findings
Edema and hemorrhage cause a change in the signal that can be differentiated from changes due to fibrous tissue replacement of muscle. This allows localization of the problem and helps to identify the type of problem.

DIAGNOSTIC PROCEDURES

Muscle Biopsy
The presence of fibrous tissue and the loss of muscle cells may be documented. Differentiating disuse atrophy from neurologic atrophy and from injury-induced scarring may be impossible without corroborating evidence.

 TREATMENT

- There is no documented evidence to support a single "best" way to treat acute muscle injuries in order to prevent fibrous contracture and adhesions. It is generally believed that immediate postinjury care should involve rest, local cold application followed within hours by heat, and passive physical therapy (movement). It would be inappropriate to hospitalize or cage a recently injured animal for muscle problems unless surgical repair is planned. Light or non–weight bearing activity would be appropriate for an extended period of time (4–6 weeks). Analgesics and antiinflammatory drugs would be recommended for several days to a week. Surgery may be performed within a few days of the injury to repair obvious, acute muscle rupture that results in a separation of the uninjured muscle segments. An essential part of muscle repair is effective

MUSCLE RUPTURE (MUSCLE TEAR)

tension relief for the injured muscle so that healing can occur without disruption as function returns. Internal or external orthopedic devices may be necessary to provide effective tension relief. Owners should be made aware of the possibility of scar-related problems affecting the patient's gait in the long term.

- Once the muscle injury becomes chronic and associated with contracture or adhesions, treatment is aimed at function salvage. Surgical release of the adhesions or fibrous tissue bands is often accompanied by instantaneous symptomatic relief. The prevention of re-adhesion and progressive contracture is much less rewarding.
- Specific muscle injuries have widely disparate prognoses. Infraspinatus contracture responds well to surgical excision of the tendon of insertion. Gracilis contracture has a 100% recurrence rate after surgical resection. Quadriceps contracture has a similarly dismal failure rate after surgery.
- Muscle injuries that have healed in an elongated state have a better prognosis for surgical improvement of function than contracted muscles. The most common elongation injury affects the muscles of the Achilles group. Hock hyperflexion can be surgically reconstructed to return these animals to relatively normal function. This is usually accomplished by shortening the Achilles tendon rather than the injured muscle or musculotendinous junction.

 MEDICATIONS

DRUG(S)
None are specific. Antiinflammatory drugs may be indicated in acute situations.

CONTRAINDICATIONS/
POSSIBLE INTERACTIONS
Immobilization of the injured muscle in a position that allows adhesions to develop to nearby bone will often result in "tie down" contractures.

FOLLOW-UP

PATIENT MONITORING
Repetitive range of motion monitoring

PREVENTION/AVOIDANCE
Early inflammation control and non–weight bearing passive physical therapy may be beneficial.

POSSIBLE COMPLICATIONS
Contracture of the muscle and fibrous replacement of muscle tissue

EXPECTED COURSE AND PROGNOSIS
Specific to the muscle and the type of injury.

MISCELLANEOUS

ASSOCIATED CONDITIONS
Joint hypermobility, angular limb deformities, flexion/extension joint abnormalities

AGE-RELATED FACTORS
Growth plate fractures in young dogs are associated with quadriceps contracture.

ABBREVIATIONS
- CT = computed tomography
- MRI = magnetic resonance imaging

Suggested Reading
Vaughan LC. Muscle and tendon injuries in dogs. J Small Anim Pract 20:711–736, 1979.

Author: Peter K. Shires
Consulting Editor: Peter K. Shires

Myasthenia Gravis

BASICS

DEFINITION
A disorder of neuromuscular transmission characterized by muscular weakness and excessive fatigability

PATHOPHYSIOLOGY
Transmission failure at the neuromuscular junction—results from structural or functional abnormalities of the nicotinic AChRs (congenital form) and from autoantibody-mediated destruction of AChRs and postsynaptic membranes (acquired form)

SYSTEMS AFFECTED
- Neuromuscular—result of abnormalities or destruction of AChRs
- Respiratory—may find aspiration pneumonia secondary to megaesophagus

GENETICS
- Congenital familial forms—Jack Russell terriers, springer spaniels, smooth fox terriers; autosomal recessive mode of inheritance
- Acquired—as with other autoimmune diseases, requires appropriate genetic background for disease to occur; multifactorial, involving environmental, infectious, and hormonal influences

INCIDENCE/PREVALENCE
- Congenital—rare
- Acquired—not uncommon in dogs; rare in cats

GEOGRAPHIC DISTRIBUTION
Worldwide

SIGNALMENT

Species
Dogs and cats

Skeletal Anatomy
(Lateral view)

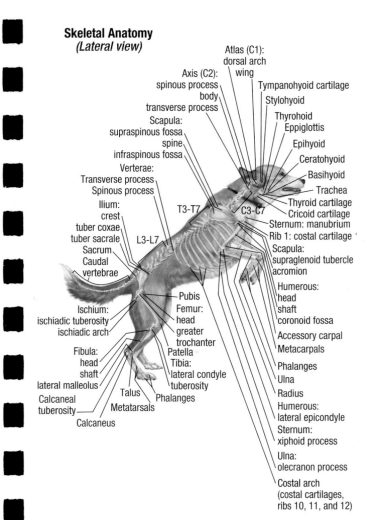

FIGURE 1.

Skeletal Anatomy
(Cranial view)

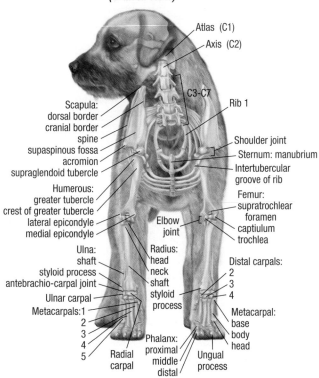

Atlas (C1)

Axis (C2)

C3-C7

Rib 1

Scapula:
dorsal border
cranial border
spine
supaspinous fossa
acromion
supraglendoid tubercle

Shoulder joint

Sternum: manubrium

Intertubercular
groove of rib

Humerous:
greater tubercle
crest of greater tubercle
lateral epicondyle
medial epicondyle

Femur:
supratrochlear
foramen
captiulum
trochlea

Elbow
joint

Ulna:
shaft
styloid process
antebrachio-carpal joint

Radius:
head
neck
shaft
styloid
process

Distal carpals:
2
3
4

Ulnar carpal

Metacarpals:1
2
3
4
5

Metacarpal:
base
body
head

Radial
carpal

Phalanx:
proximal
middle
distal

Ungual
process

FIGURE 2.

Skull
(Lateral view)

M: Molar teeth
P: Premolar teeth

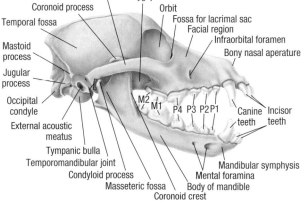

Zygomatic bone
Coronoid process
Temporal fossa
Mastoid process
Jugular process
Occipital condyle
External acoustic meatus
Tympanic bulla
Temporomandibular joint
Condyloid process
Masseteric fossa
Pterygopalatine fossa
Orbit
Fossa for lacrimal sac
Facial region
Infraorbital foramen
Bony nasal aperature
M2 M1 P4 P3 P2 P1
Canine teeth
Incisor teeth
Mandibular symphysis
Mental foramina
Body of mandible
Coronoid crest

FIGURE 3.

Skull
(Ventral view, mandible removed)

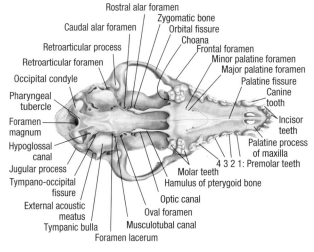

Rostral alar foramen
Zygomatic bone
Caudal alar foramen
Orbital fissure
Choana
Retroarticular process
Frontal foramen
Retroarticular foramen
Minor palatine foramen
Occipital condyle
Major palatine foramen
Palatine fissure
Pharyngeal tubercle
Canine tooth
Foramen magnum
Incisor teeth
Hypoglossal canal
Palatine process of maxilla
Jugular process
4 3 2 1: Premolar teeth
Tympano-occipital fissure
Molar teeth
External acoustic meatus
Hamulus of pterygoid bone
Tympanic bulla
Optic canal
Oval foramen
Musculotubal canal
Foramen lacerum

FIGURE 4.

3

Hip Dysplasia and Osteoarthritis

Hip Dysplasia is a term used to describe any condition which brings about abnormal development of the hip joint, resulting in osteoarthritis. As a result of joint laxity, there is complete or partial separation between the femoral head and the acetabulum (a process known as luxation or subluxation, respectively). This separation leads to abnormal wear and erosion of the joint. Eventually there is flattening of the femoral head, shallow development of the acetabulum, and formation of osteophytes (bone spurs) along the edge of the joint.

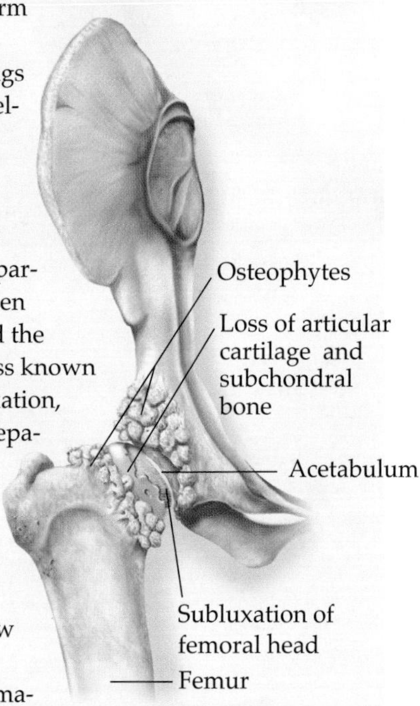

Osteophytes

Loss of articular cartilage and subchondral bone

Acetabulum

Subluxation of femoral head

Femur

FIGURE 5.

Osteochondritis Dissecans
(OCD)

OCD occurs when growing cartilage becomes thicker than normal, preventing penetration of bone marrow vessels. Under these conditions, bone formation does not proceed normally and cracks form in the cartilage. Inflammation and irritation results when the cartilage fractures, detaches and then becomes lodged within the affected joint. Joints most commonly involved are the shoulders, knees, elbows and hocks.

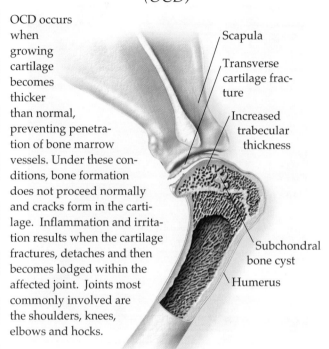

Scapula

Transverse cartilage fracture

Increased trabecular thickness

Subchondral bone cyst

Humerus

FIGURE 6.

Left Carpus and Manus
(Forepaw palmar view)

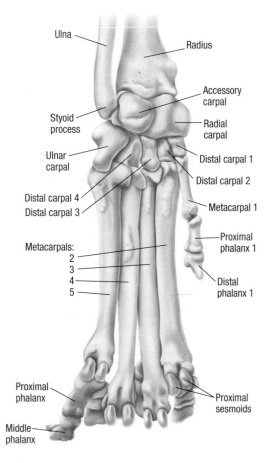

Ulna

Radius

Accessory carpal

Styoid process

Radial carpal

Ulnar carpal

Distal carpal 1

Distal carpal 2

Distal carpal 4

Distal carpal 3

Metacarpal 1

Metacarpals:
2
3
4
5

Proximal phalanx 1

Distal phalanx 1

Proximal phalanx

Proximal sesmoids

Middle phalanx

FIGURE 7.

Left Tarsus and Pes

(Hindpaw, dorsal view)   *(Hindpaw, plantar view)*

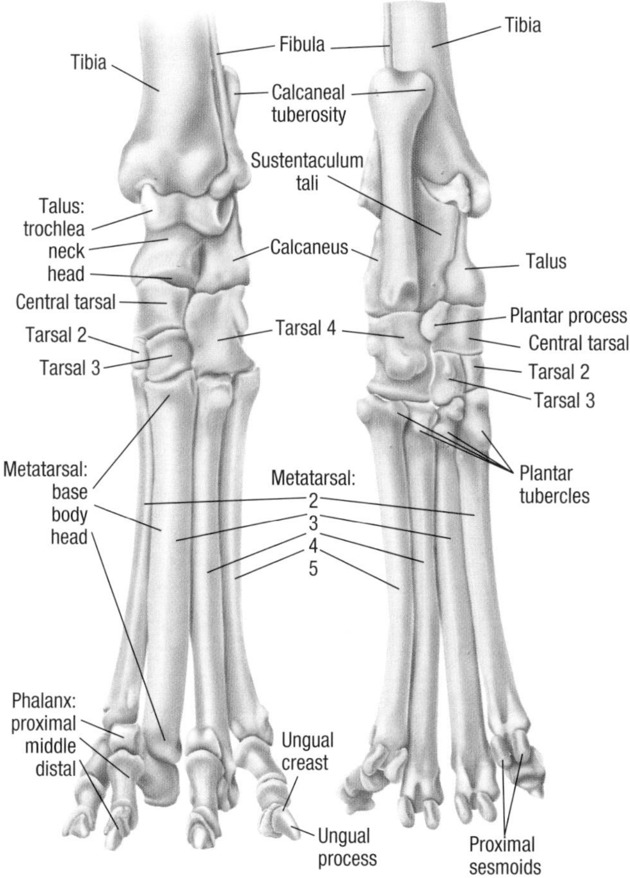

Tibia

Fibula

Tibia

Calcaneal tuberosity

Sustentaculum tali

Talus: trochlea neck head

Calcaneus

Talus

Central tarsal

Plantar process

Central tarsal

Tarsal 2
Tarsal 3

Tarsal 4

Tarsal 2

Tarsal 3

Plantar tubercles

Metatarsal: base body head

Metatarsal: 2 3 4 5

Phalanx: proximal middle distal

Ungual creast

Ungual process

Proximal sesmoids

FIGURE 8.

Muscular Anatomy
(Lateral view)

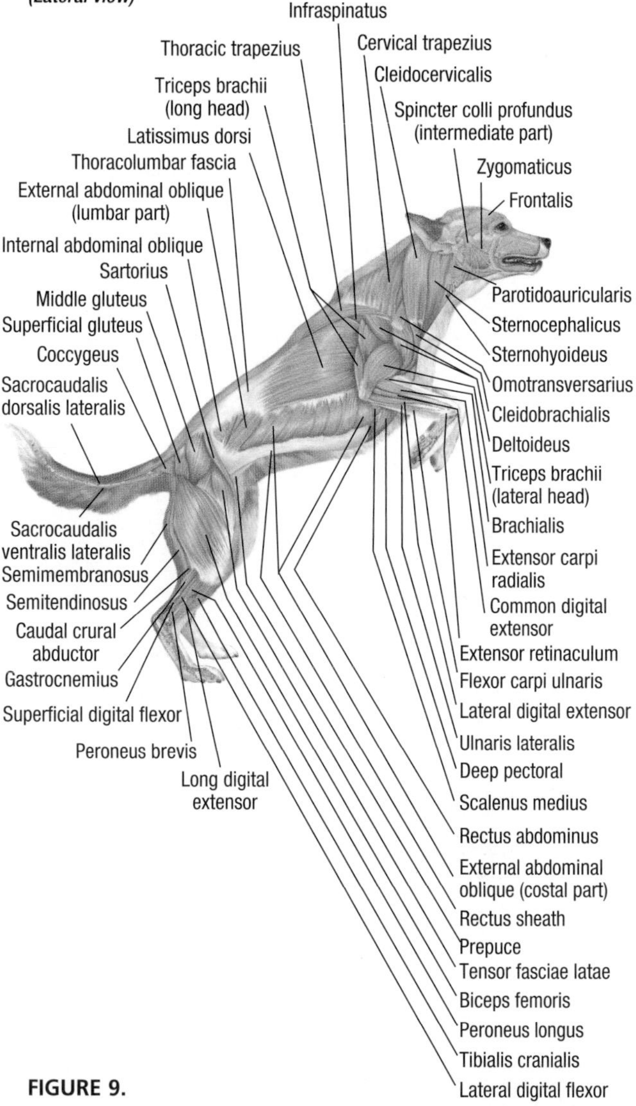

Infraspinatus
Thoracic trapezius
Cervical trapezius
Cleidocervicalis
Triceps brachii (long head)
Spincter colli profundus (intermediate part)
Latissimus dorsi
Thoracolumbar fascia
Zygomaticus
External abdominal oblique (lumbar part)
Frontalis
Internal abdominal oblique
Sartorius
Parotidoauricularis
Middle gluteus
Sternocephalicus
Superficial gluteus
Sternohyoideus
Coccygeus
Omotransversarius
Sacrocaudalis dorsalis lateralis
Cleidobrachialis
Deltoideus
Triceps brachii (lateral head)
Brachialis
Sacrocaudalis ventralis lateralis
Extensor carpi radialis
Semimembranosus
Common digital extensor
Semitendinosus
Extensor retinaculum
Caudal crural abductor
Flexor carpi ulnaris
Gastrocnemius
Lateral digital extensor
Superficial digital flexor
Ulnaris lateralis
Deep pectoral
Peroneus brevis
Scalenus medius
Long digital extensor
Rectus abdominus
External abdominal oblique (costal part)
Rectus sheath
Prepuce
Tensor fasciae latae
Biceps femoris
Peroneus longus
Tibialis cranialis
Lateral digital flexor

FIGURE 9.

8

Muscular Anatomy
(Cranial view)

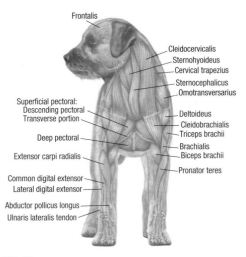

Frontalis

Cleidocervicalis
Sternohyoideus
Cervical trapezius
Sternocephalicus
Omotransversarius

Superficial pectoral:
Descending pectoral
Transverse portion

Deltoideus
Cleidobrachialis
Triceps brachii

Deep pectoral

Brachialis
Biceps brachii

Extensor carpi radialis

Pronator teres

Common digital extensor
Lateral digital extensor

Abductor pollicus longus
Ulnaris lateralis tendon

FIGURE 10.

Superficial Muscles of the Head
(Lateral view)

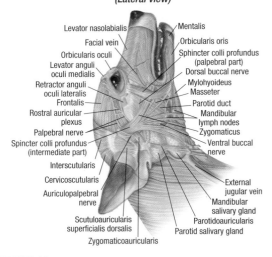

Levator nasolabialis
Facial vein
Orbicularis oculi
Levator anguli
oculi medialis
Retractor anguli
oculi lateralis
Frontalis
Rostral auricular
plexus
Palpebral nerve
Spincter colli profundus
(intermediate part)
Interscutularis
Cervicoscutularis
Auriculopalpebral
nerve
Scutuloauricularis
superficialis dorsalis
Zygomaticoauricularis

Mentalis
Orbicularis oris
Sphincter colli profundus
(palpebral part)
Dorsal buccal nerve
Mylohyoideus
Masseter
Parotid duct
Mandibular
lymph nodes
Zygomaticus
Ventral buccal
nerve
External
jugular vein
Mandibular
salivary gland
Parotidoauricularis
Parotid salivary gland

FIGURE 11.

Deep Muscles of the Head
(Lateral view)

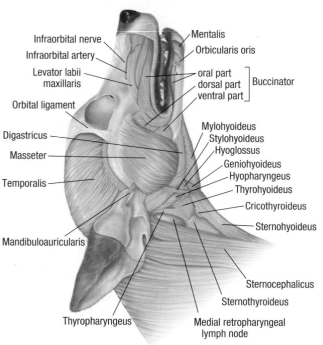

Infraorbital nerve
Infraorbital artery
Levator labii maxillaris
Orbital ligament
Digastricus
Masseter
Temporalis
Mandibuloauricularis

Mentalis
Orbicularis oris
oral part
dorsal part } Buccinator
ventral part
Mylohyoideus
Stylohyoideus
Hyoglossus
Geniohyoideus
Hyopharyngeus
Thyrohyoideus
Cricothyroideus
Sternohyoideus

Sternocephalicus
Sternothyroideus

Thyropharyngeus
Medial retropharyngeal lymph node

FIGURE 12.

Skeletal Anatomy
(Lateral view)

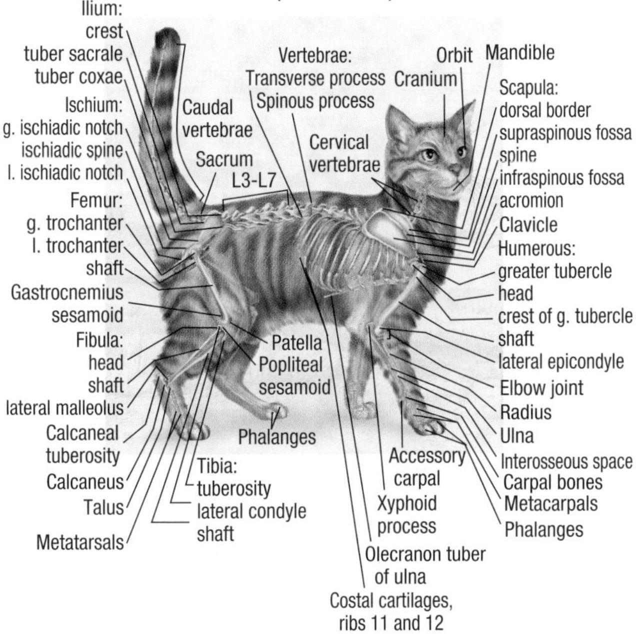

Ilium:
crest
tuber sacrale
tuber coxae
Ischium:
g. ischiadic notch
ischiadic spine
l. ischiadic notch
Femur:
g. trochanter
l. trochanter
shaft
Gastrocnemius
sesamoid
Fibula:
head
shaft
lateral malleolus
Calcaneal
tuberosity
Calcaneus
Talus
Metatarsals

Caudal
vertebrae
Sacrum
L3-L7

Vertebrae:
Transverse process
Spinous process
Cervical
vertebrae

Patella
Popliteal
sesamoid
Phalanges

Tibia:
tuberosity
lateral condyle
shaft

Orbit   Mandible
Cranium

Scapula:
dorsal border
supraspinous fossa
spine
infraspinous fossa
acromion
Clavicle
Humerous:
greater tubercle
head
crest of g. tubercle
shaft
lateral epicondyle
Elbow joint
Radius
Ulna
Interosseous space
Carpal bones
Metacarpals
Phalanges

Accessory
carpal
Xyphoid
process

Olecranon tuber
of ulna
Costal cartilages,
ribs 11 and 12

FIGURE 13.

Skeletal Anatomy
(Ventral view)

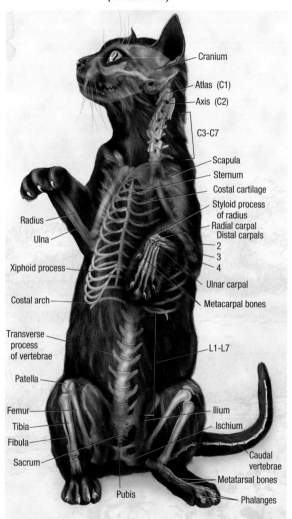

Cranium

Atlas (C1)

Axis (C2)

C3-C7

Scapula

Sternum

Costal cartilage

Styloid process of radius

Radial carpal

Distal carpals

2

3

4

Ulnar carpal

Metacarpal bones

Radius

Ulna

Xiphoid process

Costal arch

Transverse process of vertebrae

L1-L7

Patella

Femur

Tibia

Fibula

Sacrum

Ilium

Ischium

Caudal vertebrae

Metatarsal bones

Pubis

Phalanges

FIGURE 14.

Skull
(Lateral view)

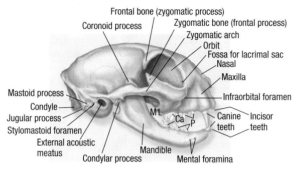

Coronoid process
Frontal bone (zygomatic process)
Zygomatic bone (frontal process)
Zygomatic arch
Orbit
Fossa for lacrimal sac
Nasal
Maxilla
Infraorbital foramen
Mastoid process
Condyle
Jugular process
Stylomastoid foramen
External acoustic meatus
Condylar process
Mandible
Mental foramina
M1
Ca
P
Canine teeth
Incisor teeth

M: molar teeth
Ca: carnassial teeth
P: premolar teeth

FIGURE 15.

Skull
(Ventral view, mandible removed)

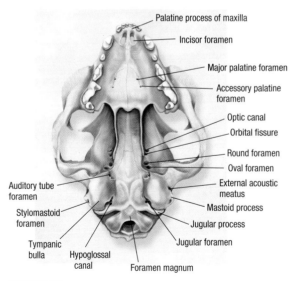

Palatine process of maxilla
Incisor foramen
Major palatine foramen
Accessory palatine foramen
Optic canal
Orbital fissure
Round foramen
Oval foramen
External acoustic meatus
Mastoid process
Jugular process
Jugular foramen
Foramen magnum
Hypoglossal canal
Tympanic bulla
Stylomastoid foramen
Auditory tube foramen

FIGURE 16.

Claw
(A: Fully retracted, B: Protruded)

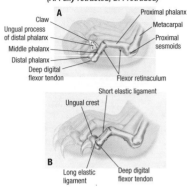

FIGURE 17.

Left Tarsus and Pes
(Hindpaw, dorsal view)   (Hindpaw, plantar view)

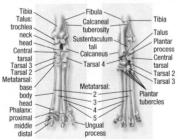

FIGURE 18.

14

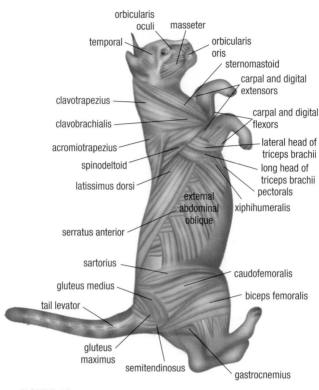

orbicularis oculi
masseter
temporal
orbicularis oris
sternomastoid
carpal and digital extensors
clavotrapezius
carpal and digital flexors
clavobrachialis
acromiotrapezius
lateral head of triceps brachii
spinodeltoid
long head of triceps brachii
latissimus dorsi
pectorals
external abdominal oblique
xiphihumeralis
serratus anterior
sartorius
caudofemoralis
gluteus medius
biceps femoralis
tail levator
gluteus maximus
semitendinosus
gastrocnemius

FIGURE 19.

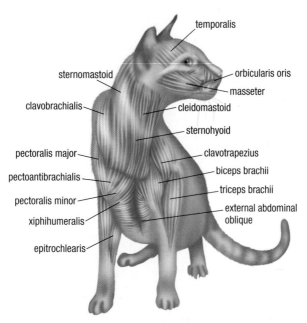

FIGURE 20.

Breed Predilections
- Congenital—Jack Russell terriers; springer spaniels; smooth fox terriers
- Acquired—several breeds: golden retrievers; German shepherds; Labrador retrievers; dachshunds; Scottish terriers; Akitas

Mean Age and Range
- Congenital—6–8 weeks of age
- Acquired—bimodal age of onset; dogs: 1–4 years of age and 9–13 years of age

Predominant Sex
- Congenital—none
- Acquired—may be a slight predilection for females in the young age group; none in the old age group

SIGNS

GENERAL COMMENTS
- Acquired—may have several clinical presentations ranging from focal involvement of the esophageal, pharyngeal, and extraocular muscles to acute generalized collapse
- Should be on the differential diagnosis of any dog with acquired megaesophagus or lower motor neuron weakness

Historical Findings
- Regurgitation—common; important to differentiate between vomiting and regurgitation
- Voice change
- Exercise-related weakness
- Acute collapse
- Progressive weakness

Physical Examination Findings
- Patient may look normal at rest.
- Excessive drooling, regurgitation, and repeated attempts at swallowing
- Muscle atrophy—usually not found
- Dyspnea—with aspiration pneumonia
- Fatigue or cramping—with mild exercise
- Careful neurologic examination—subtle findings: decreased or absent palpebral reflex (may be fatigable);

MYASTHENIA GRAVIS

may note a poor or absent gag reflex; spinal reflexes usually normal but fatigable (rarely absent and dog unable to support its weight)

CAUSES
- Congenital
- Immune-mediated
- Paraneoplastic

RISK FACTORS
- Appropriate genetic background
- Neoplasia—particularly thymoma
- Methimazole treatment (cats)—may result in reversible disease

 DIAGNOSIS

DIFFERENTIAL DIAGNOSIS
- Other disorders of neuromuscular transmission—tick paralysis; botulism; cholinesterase toxicity
- Acute or chronic polyneuropathies
- Polymyopathies—including polymyositis
- Diagnosis depends upon a careful history, thorough physical and neurologic examinations, and specialized laboratory testing.

CBC/BIOCHEMISTRY/URINALYSIS
- Normal
- Serum creatine kinase—usually normal; may be elevated with polymyositis associated with concurrent thymoma

OTHER LABORATORY TESTS
- Serum AChR antibody titer—diagnostic for acquired form
- Thyroid and adrenal function—may see abnormalities associated with acquired form

IMAGING
Thoracic radiographs—megaesophagus; cranial mediastinal mass

DIAGNOSTIC PROCEDURES
- Ultrasound-guided biopsy of cranial mediastinal mass—may support diagnosis of thymoma

- Dramatic increase in muscle strength after administration of edrophonium chloride (0.1 mg/kg IV)—may see false-negative and false-positive responses
- Decreased or absent palpebral reflex—may return after edrophonium chloride administration
- Electrophysiologic evaluation—necessity questionable with increased availability of AChR antibody testing; many patients with acquired form are poor anesthetic risks.
- Electrocardiogram—with bradycardia; third-degree heart block was recently documented in some patients with acquired disease.

PATHOLOGIC FINDINGS

Biopsy of a cranial mediastinal mass may reveal thymoma, thymic hyperplasia, or thymic atrophy.

 TREATMENT

APPROPRIATE HEALTH CARE

- Inpatient—until adequate dosages of anticholinesterase drugs are achieved
- Aspiration pneumonia—may require intensive care
- Gastrostomy tube—may be required if patient is unable to eat or drink without significant regurgitation

NURSING CARE

- Oxygen therapy, intensive antibiotic therapy, intravenous fluid therapy, and supportive care—generally required for aspiration pneumonia
- Nutritional maintenance with a gastrostomy tube—multiple feedings of a high-calorie diet; good hygiene care

ACTIVITY

Self-limited owing to the severity of muscle weakness and extent of aspiration pneumonia

DIET

May try different consistencies of food—gruel; hard food; soft food; evaluate what is best tolerated

CLIENT EDUCATION

- Warn client that, although the disease is treatable, most patients require months of special feeding and medication.

MYASTHENIA GRAVIS

- Inform client that a dedicated owner is important to a favorable outcome for acquired myasthenia.

SURGICAL CONSIDERATIONS
- Cranial mediastinal mass—thymoma
- Before attempting surgical removal, stabilize patient with anticholinesterase drugs and treat aspiration pneumonia.
- Weakness may not be seen initially.
- Suspected thymoma—test all patients for acquired disease before surgery.

 MEDICATIONS

DRUG(S) OF CHOICE
- Anticholinesterase drugs—prolong the action of acetylcholine at the neuromuscular junction; pyridostigmine bromide syrup (Mestinon syrup) at 1–3 mg/kg PO q8–12h diluted half and half in water
- Corticosteroids—0.5 mg/kg q24h; initiated if there is a poor response to pyridostigmine or if there is no response to the edrophonium chloride challenge

CONTRAINDICATIONS
Avoid drugs that may reduce the safety margin of neuromuscular transmission—aminoglycoside antibiotics; antiarrhythmic agents; phenothiazines; anesthetics; narcotics; muscle relaxants; magnesium

PRECAUTIONS
- Avoid large volumes of barium for evaluating megaesophagus.
- Large air-filled esophagus seen on survey radiographs—barium study not indicated
- Avoid immunosuppressive dosages of prednisone—may worsen muscle weakness
- Avoid unnecessary vaccinations.

POSSIBLE INTERACTIONS
N/A

ALTERNATIVE DRUG(S)
Azathroprine—2.0 mg/kg PO through gastrostomy tube q24h. Taper to q48h when clinical remission of the disease.

FOLLOW-UP

PATIENT MONITORING
- Return of muscle strength should be evident.
- Thoracic radiographs—evaluated every 4–6 weeks for resolution of megaesophagus
- AChR antibody titers—evaluated every 6–8 weeks; decrease to the normal range with clinical remission

PREVENTION/AVOIDANCE
N/A

POSSIBLE COMPLICATIONS
- Aspiration pneumonia
- Respiratory arrest

EXPECTED COURSE AND PROGNOSIS
- No severe aspiration pneumonia or pharyngeal weakness—good prognosis for complete recovery; resolution usually within 4–6 months
- Thymoma present—guarded prognosis unless complete surgical removal and control of myasthenic symptoms are achieved

 MISCELLANEOUS

ASSOCIATED CONDITIONS
- Other autoimmune disorders—thyroiditis; skin disorders; hypoadrenocorticism
- Disorders of the thymus—thymoma; thymic hyperplasia
- Other neoplasias

AGE-RELATED FACTORS
Bimodal age of onset—1–4 years of age and 9–13 years of age

ZOONOTIC POTENTIAL
N/A

PREGNANCY
- Humans—weakness may improve during pregnancy but worsens after delivery; some neonates of affected

mothers have a temporary myasthenia gravis–like weakness that lasts several days to weeks that is due to in utero transfer of autoantibodies from the mother.
• Documented in dogs after whelping

SEE ALSO
• Chapters covering autoimmune diseases
• Megaesophagus

ABBREVIATION
AChR = acetylcholine receptor

Suggested Reading

Drachman DB. Myasthenia gravis. N Eng J Med 1994;330: 1797–1810.

Shelton GD. Canine myasthenia gravis. In: Kirk WR, Bangor JD, eds. Current veterinary Therapy XI. Philadelphia: Saunders, 1992:1039–1040.

Shelton GD. Megaesophagus secondary to myasthenia gravis. In: Kirk WR, Bonagura JD, eds. Current veterinary therapy XI. Philadelphia: Saunders, 1992:580–583.

Shelton GD, Lendstrom JM. Spontaneous remission in canine myasthenia gravis: Implications for assessing human MG therapies. Neurology 2001;57:2139–2141.

Shelton GD. Myasthenia gravis and disorders of neuromuscular transmission. Vet Clin North Am 2002;31:189–200.

Author: G. Diane Shelton
Consulting Editor: Peter K. Shires

Myopathy, Focal Inflammatory—Masticatory Muscle Myositis and Extraocular Myositis

BASICS

DEFINITION
- Masticatory—focal inflammatory myopathy affecting the muscles of mastication (temporalis and masseter muscles) and sparing the limb muscles
- Extraocular—selectively affects the extraocular muscles, sparing limb and masticatory muscles

PATHOPHYSIOLOGY
- Masticatory—suspected immune-mediated cause owing to autoantibodies against type 2M fibers and a positive clinical response to immunosuppressive doses of corticosteroids
- Extraocular—suspected immune-mediated cause owing to positive clinical response to corticosteroids

SYSTEMS AFFECTED
Neuromuscular—muscles of mastication; extraocular muscles

GENETICS
- Unknown
- As with autoimmune diseases in general, the appropriate genetic background must exist.
- Extraocular—golden retrievers may have a genetic predisposition.

INCIDENCE/PREVALENCE
- Unknown
- Masticatory—not rare

GEOGRAPHIC DISTRIBUTION
Probably worldwide

MYOPATHY, FOCAL INFLAMMATORY

SIGNALMENT

Species
Dogs

Breed Predilections
- Various
- Extraocular—golden retrievers

Mean Age and Range
- No obvious age predisposition

Predominant Sex
- None obvious

SIGNS

General Comments
Masticatory—usually related to abnormalities of jaw movement and jaw pain; not a "tabletop" diagnosis; usually requires laboratory testing to confirm diagnosis

Historical Findings
- Masticatory—acute or chronic pain when opening the jaw; inability to pick up a ball or get food into the mouth; acutely swollen muscles; progressive muscle atrophy
- Extraocular—bilateral exophthalmos

Physical Examination Findings
- Masticatory—marked jaw pain with manipulation and/or trismus; acute muscle swelling with exophthalmos; muscle atrophy with enophthalmos; inability to open the jaw under anesthesia
- Extraocular—bilateral exophthalmos; impaired vision

CAUSES
Immune mediated

RISK FACTORS
- Appropriate genetic background
- Possible previous bacterial or viral infection

DIAGNOSIS

DIFFERENTIAL DIAGNOSIS
- Retro-orbital abscess—probe behind last upper molar
- Temporomandibular joint disease—radiographically abnormal joint
- Polymyositis—high serum creatine kinase; generalized EMG abnormalities; diagnostic muscle biopsies
- Neurogenic atrophy of temporalis muscles—determined by EMG and muscle biopsy
- Atrophy of masticatory muscles from corticosteroids— history of corticosteroid use; characteristic changes on muscle biopsy

CBC/BIOCHEMISTRY/URINALYSIS
Serum creatine kinase—normal or mildly elevated

OTHER LABORATORY TESTS
- Muscle biopsy—diagnostic test of choice for masticatory disease
- Immunocytochemical assay—demonstrate autoantibodies against masticatory muscle type 2M fibers; negative in polymyositis and extraocular disease

IMAGING
- Radiography of the temporomandibular joints
- Orbital sonogram—for extraorbital disease; demonstrate swollen extraocular muscles
- MRI—for demonstration of inflammation in muscles

DIAGNOSTIC PROCEDURES
EMG—differentiate between extraocular disease and polymyositis; abnormal masticatory muscles in masticatory myositis only; generalized abnormalities in polymyositis

PATHOLOGIC FINDINGS

Masticatory
- Swelling or atrophy of the masticatory muscles
- Biopsy specimen—may see myofiber necrosis, phagocytosis, mononuclear cell infiltration with a multifocal and

perivascular distribution; may see myofiber atrophy and fibrosis with chronic condition; eosinophils rare

Extraocular
Mononuclear cell infiltration—restricted to extraocular muscles

 TREATMENT

APPROPRIATE HEALTH CARE
Outpatient

NURSING CARE
Gastrostomy tube—may be required with severe restrictions in jaw mobility; requires good hygiene and supportive care

ACTIVITY
N/A

DIET
Masticatory—may require liquid food or gruel until jaw mobility is regained; may need a gastric feeding tube to facilitate fluid and caloric intake

CLIENT EDUCATION
- Warn client that long-term corticosteroid therapy may be required.
- Inform client that residual muscle atrophy and restricted jaw movement may occur with chronic masticatory disease.

SURGICAL CONSIDERATIONS
Not indicated

 MEDICATIONS

DRUG(S) OF CHOICE
Coricosteroids—immunosuppressive dosages, tapered as jaw mobility, swelling, and serum creatine kinase return to normal; maintained at lowest alternate-day dosage that prevents restricted jaw mobility; treated for a minimum of 6 months

CONTRAINDICATIONS
N/A

PRECAUTIONS
- Corticosteroids—watch for infection and undesirable side effects.
- Clinical signs may recur if treatment is stopped too soon.

POSSIBLE INTERACTIONS
N/A

ALTERNATIVE DRUG(S)
Intolerable side effects of corticosteroids—institute a lower dose of corticosteroids and combine with another drug (e.g., azathioprine).

 FOLLOW-UP

PATIENT MONITORING
- Masticatory—return of jaw mobility and decreased serum creatine kinase
- Extraocular—decreased swelling of extraocular muscles

PREVENTION/AVOIDANCE
N/A

POSSIBLE COMPLICATIONS
- Corticosteroids—undesirable side effects
- Recurrence of clinical signs—treatment stopped too early
- Poor clinical response—inadequate dosages of corticosteroids
- Restrictive strabismus (extraocular myositis)

EXPECTED COURSE AND PROGNOSIS
- Masticatory—jaw mobility should return to normal unless the condition is chronic and severe fibrosis develops; good prognosis if treated early with adequate dosages of corticosteroids
- Extraocular—good response to corticosteroids; good prognosis

127

MYOPATHY, FOCAL INFLAMMATORY

 MISCELLANEOUS

ASSOCIATED CONDITIONS
Other concurrent autoimmune disorders

AGE-RELATED FACTORS
N/A

ZOONOTIC POTENTIAL
N/A

PREGNANCY
Unknown

SYNONYMS
- Eosinophilic myositis
- Atrophic myositis

SEE ALSO
- Myopathy, Generalized Inflammatory– Polymyositis and Dermatomyositis
- Myopathy, Noninflammatory–Endocrine

ABBREVIATIONS
- EMG = electromyogram
- MRI = magnetic resonance imaging

Suggested Reading

Allgoewer I, Blair M, Basher T, Davidson Metal. Extraocular myositis and restrictive strabismus in 10 dogs. Vet Ophth 2003;21–26.

Carpenter JL, Schmidt GM, Moore FM, et al. Canine bilateral extraocular polymyositis. Vet Pathol 1989;26:510–512.

Orvis JS, Cardinet GH III. Canine muscle fiber types and susceptibility of masticatory muscles to myositis. Muscle Nerve 1981;4:354–359.

Podell M. Inflammatory myopathies. Vet Clin North Am 2002;31:147–167.

Shelton GD, Cardinet GH III, Bandman E. Canine masticatory muscle disorders: a clinicopathological and immuno-chemical study of 29 cases. Muscle Nerve 1987;10: 753–766.

Shelton GD. Canine masticatory muscle disorders. In Kirk
RW, ed. Current veterinary therapy X. Philadelphia:
Saunders, 1989;816–819.

Author: G. Diane Shelton
Consulting Editor: Peter K. Shires

Myopathy, Generalized Inflammatory— Polymyositis and Dermatomyositis

 BASICS

DEFINITION
- Polymyositis—a condition in which skeletal muscles are damaged by a nonsuppurative inflammatory process dominated by lymphocytic infiltration
- Dermatomyositis—polymyositis is associated with characteristic skin lesions

PATHOPHYSIOLOGY
- Inflammation of skeletal muscles—results in muscle weakness, myalgia, and atrophy
- Muscle inflammation—may be a result of immune-mediated, infectious, or paraneoplastic disorders; may be a sequela to certain drug therapies

SYSTEMS AFFECTED
- Neuromuscular—generalized muscle involvement including masticatory and limb muscles
- Gastrointestinal—particularly the pharyngeal and esophageal muscles, because they are composed predominantly of skeletal muscle in dogs
- Skin/Exocrine—particularly if related to a generalized immune-mediated connective tissue disorder

Genetics
- Unknown
- As for autoimmune diseases in general, the appropriate genetic background must exist.
- Dermatomyositis—reported to have an autosomal dominant inheritance pattern in rough-coated collies and Shetland sheepdogs

MYOPATHY, GENERALIZED INFLAMMATORY

INCIDENCE/PREVALENCE
- Unknown
- Generalized inflammatory myopathies—not common

GEOGRAPHIC DISTRIBUTION
Probably worldwide

SIGNALMENT

Species
Dogs and rarely cats

Breed Predilections
- Polymyositis—various breeds of dogs and cats may be affected; breed-associated in Newfoundland and boxer
- Dermatomyositis—reported in rough-coated collies, Shetland sheepdogs, and Australian cattle dogs

Mean Age and Range
- Polymyositis—none obvious
- Dermatomyositis—3–5 months of age

Predominant Sex
None obvious

SIGNS

General Comments
- Polymyositis—usually associated with a stiff-stilted gait, muscle pain, and/or muscle weakness. May see regurgitation and megaesophagus
- Elevated serum creatine kinase—supports but does not make the diagnosis of myositis
- Muscle biopsy—needed to confirm the diagnosis

Historical Findings
- Stiff-stilted gait—acute or chronic
- Muscle swelling and/or atrophy
- Generalized muscle pain
- Generalized muscle weakness and exercise intolerance
- Regurgitation of food or difficulty swallowing

Physical Examination Findings
- Pain upon palpation of muscle groups
- Generalized muscle atrophy, including the muscles of mastication

MYOPATHY, GENERALIZED INFLAMMATORY

- Gait abnormalities, including a stiff-stilted gait
- Neurologic examination—not abnormal; may be a decreased gag reflex if the pharyngeal muscles are affected
- Dermatomyositis (dogs)—typical skin lesions

CAUSES
- Immune-mediated
- Infectious—*Toxoplasma gondii; Neospora canis; Hepatozoon canis; Ehrlichia canis;* bacterial infection uncommon
- Drug-induced
- Paraneoplastic syndrome

RISK FACTORS
- Appropriate genetic background
- Possibly previous bacterial or viral infection
- Neoplasia, possibly occult

 DIAGNOSIS

DIFFERENTIAL DIAGNOSIS
- Polyarthritis—differentiated by physical examination and evaluation of joint fluid
- Noninflammatory muscle disorders—differentiated by muscle biopsy
- Polyneuropathy—differentiated by neurologic examination, electrophysiology, and muscle biopsy
- Chronic intervertebral disk disease—differentiated by physical examination and serum creatine kinase

CBC/BIOCHEMISTRY/URINALYSIS
Serum creatine kinase—variably elevated

OTHER LABORATORY TESTS
- Serum antinuclear antibody titer—may be positive in connective tissue disorders
- May see concurrent hypothyroidism

IMAGING
- Regurgitation—evaluate thoracic radiography for esophageal dilatation.

- Pharyngeal weakness—perform a dynamic study for the evaluation of the swallowing process.

DIAGNOSTIC PROCEDURES
- Muscle biopsy—single most important test for diagnosing polymyositis; sample multiple muscles, because condition may be missed if distribution is patchy
- Electromyographic evaluation—performed to determine the distribution of muscle involvement and the muscles to be biopsied; should help differentiate myopathic from neuropathic causes of muscle weakness

PATHOLOGIC FINDINGS
- Muscle swelling or atrophy
- Biopsy specimens—usually contain mononuclear cell infiltrates
- Rare neutrophils or eosinophils—may be noted
- Regenerating myofibers—may be observed
- Intramyofiber parasite cyst—rare
- Chronic condition—may see extensive myofiber atrophy and fibrosis

 TREATMENT

APPROPRIATE HEALTH CARE
Outpatient

NURSING CARE
Supportive care—may be required to prevent skin wounds and decubital ulcers in nonambulatory severely affected patients

ACTIVITY
Should increase, along with muscle strength, as muscle inflammation decreases

DIET
- Megaesophagus—may require feeding from an elevation; try foods of different consistencies.
- Severe regurgitation—may need to place a gastric feeding tube to maintain hydration and nutrition

MYOPATHY, GENERALIZED INFLAMMATORY

CLIENT EDUCATION
- Warn client that long-term immunosuppressive therapy may be required for an immune-mediated condition.
- Inform client that residual muscle atrophy may occur with chronic disease and extensive fibrosis.
- Suggest genetic counseling for familial disorders.

SURGICAL CONSIDERATIONS
Only for concurrent neoplasia.

 MEDICATIONS

DRUG(S) OF CHOICE
- Corticosteroids—immunosuppressive dosages usually result in clinical improvement of immune-mediated condition; decrease to the lowest alternate-day dosage that maintains normal creatine kinase and improved muscle strength and mobility; may require long-term therapy
- Identified infectious agent—initiate specific therapy.

CONTRAINDICATIONS
N/A

PRECAUTIONS
Corticosteroids—observe for infection and undesirable side effects; remember that chronic therapy may lead to muscle atrophy

POSSIBLE INTERACTIONS
N/A

ALTERNATIVE DRUG(S)
Intolerable side effects of corticosteroids—institute a lower dose of corticosteroids combined with another drug (e.g., azathioprine)

 FOLLOW-UP

PATIENT MONITORING
- Serum creatine kinase—periodic evaluation; if elevated, should decrease into the normal range
- Corticosteroids—side effects

PREVENTION/AVOIDANCE
N/A

POSSIBLE COMPLICATIONS
- Corticosteroids—undesirable side effects
- Recurrence of clinical signs—treatment stopped too early
- Poor clinical response—inadequate dosages of corticosteroids

EXPECTED COURSE AND PROGNOSIS
- Immune-mediated condition—good to fair prognosis
- Paraneoplastic disorder associated with occult neoplasia—guarded prognosis

 MISCELLANEOUS

ASSOCIATED CONDITIONS
- Other concurrent autoimmune disorders
- Neoplasia

AGE-RELATED FACTORS
N/A

ZOONOTIC POTENTIAL
N/A

PREGNANCY
Unknown

SEE ALSO
Myopathy, Noninflammatory–Endocrine

Suggested Reading

Hargis AM, Haupt KH, Prieur DJ, Moore MP. A skin disorder in three Shetland sheepdogs: comparison with familial canine dermatomyositis of collies. Compend Contin Educ Pract Vet 1985;7:306–318.

Kornegay JN, Gorgacz EJ, Dawe DL, et al. Polymyositis in dogs. J Am Vet Med Assoc 1980;176:431–438.

Podell M. Inflammatory myopathies. Vet Clin North Am 2002;31:147–167.

Shelton GD, Cardinet GH III. Pathophysiologic basis of canine muscle disorders. J Vet Intern Med 1987;1:36–44.

Author: G. Diane Shelton
Consulting Editor: Peter K. Shires

Myopathy, Noninflammatory– Endocrine

 BASICS

DEFINITION
Myopathies associated with various endocrinopathies (including hypothyroidism, hyperthyroidism, hypoadrenocorticism, hyperadrenocorticism) and associated with exogenous corticosteroid use (steroid myopathy)

PATHOPHYSIOLOGY

With Adrenal Dysfunction
- Glucocorticoid excess—impaired muscle protein metabolism; may accelerate degradation of myofibrillar and soluble protein in skeletal muscle; impairment of carbohydrate metabolism owing to induction of an insulin-resistant state; may note elevated ACTH levels
- Adrenal insufficiency—circulatory insufficiency; fluid and electrolyte imbalance; impaired carbohydrate metabolism

With Thyroid Disease
- Hyperthyroidism—increased mitochondrial respiration; accelerated protein degradation and lipid oxidation; glycogen depletion; impaired glucose uptake
- Hypothyroidism—impaired muscle energy metabolism by reduced glycogen breakdown, gluconeogenesis, and oxidative and glycolytic capacity; impaired insulin-stimulated carbohydrate metabolism

SYSTEMS AFFECTED
- Neuromuscular—impaired energy metabolism
- Cardiovascular—impaired energy metabolism; circulatory disorders

GENETICS
N/A

MYOPATHY, NONINFLAMMATORY–ENDOCRINE

INCIDENCE/PREVALENCE
- Exact incidence unknown
- Myopathies related to exogenous corticosteroids—common
- Myopathies associated with Cushing syndrome and hypothyroidism—not uncommon

GEOGRAPHIC DISTRIBUTION
Probably worldwide

SIGNALMENT

Species
- Dogs—steroid myopathy; weakness associated with hyperadrenocorticism and hypoadrenocorticism; hypothyroidism
- Cats—weakness associated with hyperthyroidism

Breed Predilections
Affects several breeds

MEAN AGE AND RANGE
- Steroid myopathy—dogs of any age
- Other disorders—see specific disease

Predominant Sex
None found

SIGNS

General Comments
Corticosteroid use in dogs—muscles very susceptible; muscle atrophy (particularly the masticatory muscles) is not uncommon with prolonged corticosteroid use

Historical Findings
- Muscle weakness, atrophy, and stiffness
- Regurgitation
- Dysphagia
- Dysphonia

Physical Examination Findings
- Muscle weakness, stiffness, cramping, and myalgia
- Muscle hypertrophy or atrophy
- May not note other clinical signs of an endocrine disorder

MYOPATHY, NONINFLAMMATORY–ENDOCRINE

CAUSES
- Endocrine dysfunction
- Autoimmune
- Neoplastic

RISK FACTORS
N/A

 DIAGNOSIS

DIFFERENTIAL DIAGNOSIS
- Inflammatory myopathies—distinguished by muscle biopsy
- Noninflammatory myopathies—distinguished by muscle biopsy

CBC/BIOCHEMISTRY/URINALYSIS
- Baseline testing—abnormalities consistent with endocrine disorder
- Serum creatine kinase—usually normal

OTHER LABORATORY TESTS
Thyroid and adrenal function tests—should be diagnostic

IMAGING
- Dynamic studies—evaluate pharyngeal and esophageal function; with regurgitation and dysphagia
- Cardiac evaluation—for cats with hyperthyroidism

DIAGNOSTIC PROCEDURES
- Muscle biopsy—fresh frozen sections
- Electromyography

PATHOLOGIC FINDINGS
- Hyperadrenocorticism and steroid myopathies—selective atrophy of type 2 muscle fibers; may see lobulated or ragged-red fibers with associated myotonia
- Hypoadrenocorticism—normal
- Hyperthyroidism (cats)—unknown if pathologic abnormalities occur within muscle
- Hypothyroidism—atrophy of type 2 fibers; may see an increase in type 1 fibers; may see PAS-positive deposits and nemaline rods in type 2 fibers

TREATMENT

APPROPRIATE HEALTH CARE
Depends on specific endocrine disorder

NURSING CARE
Support bandaging, wound management (decubital ulcers), and physical therapy—with musculoskeletal manifestations

ACTIVITY
- Clinical corticosteroid myopathy (humans)—inactivity worsens condition; increased muscle activity may partially prevent atrophy.
- Physical therapy—may help prevent and treat muscle weakness and wasting in dogs receiving glucocorticoids

DIET
- Regurgitation and megaesophagus—feed from an elevation.
- Dysphagia and esophageal dilation—give food with the best-tolerated consistency.
- Gastric feeding tube—if oral feeding is not tolerated

CLIENT EDUCATION
Depends on specific endocrine disorder

SURGICAL CONSIDERATIONS
Removal of neoplasia

 MEDICATIONS

DRUG(S) OF CHOICE
- Depend on specific endocrine disorder
- Corticosteroid myopathy—decrease corticosteroid dosage to the lowest possible level; use a nonfluorinated corticosteroid and alternate-day dosing.
- Intramyofiber lipid storage with steroid myopathy—L-carnitine (50 mg/kg q12h) may improve muscle strength.

CONTRAINDICATIONS
N/A

PRECAUTIONS
Depend on specific endocrine disorder

MYOPATHY, NONINFLAMMATORY–ENDOCRINE

POSSIBLE INTERACTIONS
N/A

ALTERNATIVE DRUG(S)
Fluorinated corticosteroids, triamcinolone, betamethasone, and dexamethasone—most likely to produce muscle weakness; use an equivalent dose of another corticosteroid.

 FOLLOW-UP

PATIENT MONITORING
- Depends on specific endocrine disorder
- Steroid myopathy—should note return of muscle strength and mass with decreased steroid use

PREVENTION/AVOIDANCE
N/A

POSSIBLE COMPLICATIONS
Depend on specific endocrine disorders

EXPECTED COURSE AND PROGNOSIS
- Myotonia associated with hyperadrenocorticism—poor prognosis for resolution
- Steroid myopathy—good prognosis for return of muscle strength and mass; recovery may take weeks
- Hypothyroid myopathy—improvement in muscle pain and stiffness common
- Hyperthyroidism (cats)—good prognosis for return of muscle strength following return to euthyroid state
- Hypoadrenocorticism—good prognosis for return of muscle strength
- Dysphagia and regurgitation—may resolve with adequate treatment

 MISCELLANEOUS

ASSOCIATED CONDITIONS
- May note multiple endocrinopathies
- Hypothyroidism (dogs)—concurrent myasthenia gravis

AGE-RELATED FACTORS
N/A

ZOONOTIC POTENTIAL
N/A

PREGNANCY
Unknown

ABBREVIATIONS
- ACTH = adrenocorticotropic hormone
- PAS = periodic acid–Schiff

Suggested Reading

Jaggy A, Oliver JE, Ferguson DC, et al. Neurological manifestations of hypothyroidism: a retrospective study of 29 cases. J Vet Intern Med 1994;8:328–330.

LeCouteur RA, Dow SW, Sisson AF. Metabolic and endocrine myopathies of dogs and cats. Semin Vet Med Surg Small Anim 1989;4:146–155.

Platt SR. Neuromuscular complications in endocrine and metabolic disorders. Vet Clin North Am 2002;31:125–146.

Shelton GD, Cardinet GH III. Pathophysiologic basis of canine muscle disorders. J Vet Intern Med 1987;1:36–44.

Author: G. Diane Shelton
Consulting Editor: Peter K. Shires

Myopathy, Noninflammatory— Hereditary Labrador Retriever

 BASICS

OVERVIEW
- An inherited progressive and degenerative generalized myopathy of Labrador retrievers
- Simple autosomal recessive mode of inheritance
- Pathophysiologic mechanism(s) unknown
- Histologic examination of muscle—more typical of a neurogenic than a myopathic cause; no morphologic changes in the CNS or peripheral nerves identified

SIGNALMENT
- Occurs in black and yellow Labrador retrievers
- Age of onset—variable (6 weeks to 7 months); most common at 3–4 months
- Affects males and females

SIGNS
- Severity ranges from stilted gait to muscle weakness, bunny hopping pelvic limb gait, ventroflexion of the neck, arched back, and abnormal joint posture (cow-hocked stance, hyperextended carpi)
- Worsen with exercise, excitement, and cold weather
- Patient may collapse with forced exercise.
- Some improvement with rest
- Generalized muscle atrophy—mild to severe
- Atrophy of proximal limb and masticatory muscles often most prominent
- Tendon reflexes—normal, hypoactive, or absent
- Occasionally, patients become recumbent or develop megaesophagus.

CAUSE & RISK FACTORS
Autosomal recessive mode of inheritance

 DIAGNOSIS

DIFFERENTIAL DIAGNOSIS
- With little muscle atrophy—exercise intolerance may mimic signs of myasthenia gravis or cardiac or orthopedic disease.
- With marked muscle atrophy—consider other myopathies (infectious, immune-mediated, metabolic, congenital) and generalized lower motor neuron disorders.

CBC/BIOCHEMISTRY/URINALYSIS
Creatine kinase—normal or mildly or moderately elevated

OTHER LABORATORY TESTS
N/A

IMAGING
N/A

DIAGNOSTIC PROCEDURES
- EMG—spontaneous activity, including complex repetitive discharges, especially in proximal limb and masticatory muscles; may reveal no abnormalities with mild disease
- Muscle histology—reveals variation in fiber size, angular atrophy of both type 1 and 2 myofibers, grouped atrophy, increase in central nuclei, muscle degeneration and regeneration, and fibrosis; may note deficiency or increase in type 2 myofibers

 TREATMENT

- None specific
- Avoid cold, because it exacerbates clinical signs.
- Discourage breeding of affected animals.
- Do not repeat dam–sire breedings that result in affected offspring.

143

MEDICATIONS

DRUG(S)
Diazepam may be beneficial.

CONTRAINDICATIONS/POSSIBLE INTERACTIONS
None known

 FOLLOW-UP

- Clinical signs generally stabilize.
- Mild disease—may be an acceptable pet; may show some improvement in exercise tolerance
- Aspiration pneumonia—a risk with megaesophagus

 MISCELLANEOUS

ASSOCIATED CONDITIONS
N/A

AGE-RELATED FACTORS
N/A

ZOONOTIC POTENTIAL
N/A

PREGNANCY
N/A

ABBREVIATION
EMG = electromyography

Suggested Reading
McKerrell RE, Braud KG. Hereditary myopathy of Labrador retrievers. In: Kirk RW, Bonagura JD, eds. Current veterinary therapy X. Philadelphia: Saunders, 1989:820–821.

Author: Georgina Child
Consulting Editor: Peter K. Shires

Myopathy, Noninflammatory– Hereditary Myotonia

BASICS

OVERVIEW
- Myopathy characterized by persistent contraction of muscle fibers on initiation of movement or when stimulated to contract
- May affect all skeletal muscles
- Congenital or acquired
- Congenital—may be associated with abnormal chloride conductance of muscle membrane

SIGNALMENT
- Congenital—described in young chow chows; rarely seen in other dog breeds
- Acquired—all breeds potentially susceptible
- Reported in cats

SIGNS
Historical Findings
- Difficulty rising
- Stiffness after rest
- May note dyspnea, dysphagia, and/or regurgitation
- May improve with exercise
- Exacerbated by cold

PHYSICAL EXAMINATION FINDINGS
- Hypertrophy of proximal limb muscles, neck muscles, and tongue
- Abduction of thoracic limbs
- Bunny-hopping pelvic limb gait
- Patient may fall and remain rigid in lateral recumbency for short periods.

HEREDITARY MYOTONIA

CAUSES & RISK FACTORS
Chow chows—suspected autosomal recessive mode of inheritance

 DIAGNOSIS

DIFFERENTIAL DIAGNOSIS
Other myopathies—distinguished by signalment and clinical and electromyographic findings

CBC/BIOCHEMISTRY/URINALYSIS
Creatine kinase—may be slightly elevated

OTHER LABORATORY TESTS
N/A

IMAGING
N/A

DIAGNOSTIC PROCEDURES
- Percussion of muscles and tongue in conscious and anesthetized dogs—causes sustained dimpling
- Electromyography—reveals multifocal or generalized high-frequency discharges that wax and wane in amplitude and frequency (dive bomber–sounding potentials) and that are increased after muscle percussion

PATHOLOGIC FINDINGS
- Muscle histology—shows mild changes (e.g., some angular atrophy, central nuclei, variation in fiber size)

 TREATMENT

- None specific
- Discourage activities that result in hyperventilation.
- Avoid cold.
- Anesthesia (induction and recovery)—possible risk of respiratory obstruction owing to adduction of vocal cords or regurgitation

MEDICATIONS

DRUG(S)
Membrane-stabilizing drugs—procainamide and quinidine; may decrease severity of clinical signs

CONTRAINDICATIONS/POSSIBLE INTERACTIONS
None

FOLLOW-UP

PREVENTION/AVOIDANCE
- Chow chows—inherited condition; advise owner regarding breeding.
- Discourage breeding of affected animals.
- Do not repeat dam–sire breedings that resulted in affected offspring.

POSSIBLE COMPLICATIONS
Respiratory obstruction and/or aspiration of regurgitated food—may be life-threatening; advise owners of the clinical symptoms and treatment.

EXPECTED COURSE AND PROGNOSIS
Prognosis guarded

MISCELLANEOUS

ASSOCIATED CONDITIONS
N/A

AGE-RELATED FACTORS
Aging—signs may stabilize or worsen.

ZOONOTIC POTENTIAL
N/A

PREGNANCY
N/A

HEREDITARY MYOTONIA

Suggested Reading

Amann JF, Tomlinson J, Hankison JK. Myotonia in a chow chow. J Am Vet Med Assoc 1985;187:415–417.

Duncan ID, Griffiths IR. Myotonia in the dog. In: Kirk RW, ed. Current veterinary therapy VIII. Philadelphia: Saunders, 1983:686–689.

Hill SL, Shelton GD, Lemehan TM. Myotonia in a cocker spaniel. J Am Anim Hosp Assoc 1995;31:506–509.

Honhold N, Smith DA. Myotonia in the Great Dane, Vet Rec 1986;119:162.

Shires PK, Nafe LA, Hulsie DA. Myotonia in a Staffordshire terrier. J Am Vet Med Assoc 1983;183(2):229–232.

Toll J, Copper B, Altschul M. Congenital myotonia in 2 domestic cats. J Vet Intern Med 1998;12:116–119.

Vite CH, Melniczel J, Patterson D. Congenital myotonic myopathy in the miniature schnauzer: an autosomal recessive trait. Hered 1999;90(5):578–580.

Author: Georgina Child
Consulting Editor: Peter K. Shires

Myopathy, Noninflammatory— Hereditary Scotty Cramp

 BASICS

OVERVIEW
- Inherited neurologic disorder in Scottish terriers characterized by episodic muscle hypertonicity or cramping
- Not associated with any morphologic changes in muscle, peripheral nerve, or the CNS
- Thought to be the result of a disorder in serotonin metabolism within the CNS
- Similar condition reported in young Dalmatians and Labrador retrievers—may be result of low numbers of neurotransmitter glycine receptors in the CNS

SIGNALMENT
- Young Scottish terriers, typically <1 year of age
- No known sex predilection

SIGNS
- Normal at rest and on initial exercise
- Further exercise or excitement—abduction of the thoracic limbs; arching of the lumbar spine; stiffening or overflexion of the pelvic limbs (goose-stepping gait)
- Patient may fall, with tail and pelvic limbs flexed tightly against the body
- Respiration—may cease for a short time
- Facial muscles—may be contracted
- No loss of consciousness
- Severity varies
- Episodes—may last up to 30 min

CAUSES & RISK FACTORS
Inherited condition with probable recessive mode of transmission

HEREDITARY SCOTTY CRAMP

 DIAGNOSIS

DIFFERENTIAL DIAGNOSIS
Seizure disorder—distinguished on basis of family history, typical clinical signs with no loss of consciousness, and induction of signs with serotonin antagonists

CBC/BIOCHEMISTRY/URINALYSIS
Normal

OTHER LABORATORY TESTS
N/A

IMAGING
N/A

DIAGNOSTIC PROCEDURES
Clinical signs may be induced by giving the serotonin antagonist, methysergide.

 TREATMENT

Behavioral modification and/or environmental changes—eliminating triggering situations (excitement, stress); may be adequate

 MEDICATIONS

DRUG(S)
Acepromazine, diazepam, or vitamin E—may reduce the incidence and severity of episodes

CONTRAINDICATIONS/POSSIBLE INTERACTIONS
- Serotonin antagonists—increase severity of clinical signs
- Aspirin, indomethacin, phenylbutazone, Banamine (flunixin meglumine), and penicillin—may exacerbate clinical signs

FOLLOW-UP

PATIENT MONITORING
Nonprogressive

PREVENTION/AVOIDANCE
- Discourage breeding affected animals.
- Do not repeat dam–sire breedings that result in affected offspring.

EXPECTED COURSE AND PROGNOSIS
- Mild to moderate—fair to good long-term prognosis; usually acceptable disability to owners; nonprogressive
- Severe—guarded to poor prognosis

 MISCELLANEOUS

ASSOCIATED CONDITIONS
N/A

AGE-RELATED FACTORS
N/A

ZOONOTIC POTENTIAL
N/A

PREGNANCY
N/A

Suggested Reading
Meyers KM, Clemmons RM. Scotty cramp. In: Kirk RW, ed. Current veterinary therapy VIII. Philadelphia: Saunders, 1983:702–704.

Author: Georgina Child
Consulting Editor: Peter K. Shires

Myopathy, Noninflammatory– Hereditary X-Linked Muscular Dystrophy

 BASICS

OVERVIEW
- Inherited, progressive, and degenerative generalized myopathy with X-linked mode of inheritance
- Patients lack muscle membrane–associated protein dystrophin
- RNA processing defect—identified in golden retrievers, Irish terriers, Samoyeds, rottweilers, Belgian shepherds, and one miniature schnauzer

SIGNALMENT
- Seen primarily in neonate and young dogs
- Described in cats
- Primarily affects males
- Females—usually carriers of gene defect; homozygotes may be affected.

SIGNS

Dogs
- Golden retrievers—exercise intolerance; stilted gait; bunny-hopping pelvic limb gait; plantigrade stance; partial trismus; muscle atrophy (especially the truncal and temporalis muscles); hypertrophy of some muscles (especially the tongue); kyphosis; lordosis; drooling; dysphagia; aspiration pneumonia (due to pharyngeal and/or esophageal involvement)
- Other breeds—similar; include vomiting and megaesophagus
- Vary in severity, onset, and progression; may be seen as early as 6 weeks; tend to stabilize by 6 months
- Stunting and ineffective suckling—may be evident in younger pups

HEREDITARY X-LINKED MUSCULAR DYSTROPHY

- Cardiac failure—may occur owing to cardiomyopathy
- Severe muscle contractures
- Spinal reflexes—normal initially; may become hypoactive

Cats
- Dystrophin deficient—muscle hypertrophy; stiff gait; cervical rigidity; exercise intolerance; vomiting
- Not apparent in one cat until 21 months of age

CAUSES & RISK FACTORS
Inherited defect of the X chromosome

 DIAGNOSIS

DIFFERENTIAL DIAGNOSIS
Other inherited, infectious (protozoal), immune-mediated, or metabolic myopathies; distinguished by muscle histology and demonstration of dystrophin deficiency

CBC/BIOCHEMISTRY/URINALYSIS
Normal except for marked elevation in serum creatine kinase (may be >10,000 U/L; further increased after exercise)

OTHER LABORATORY TESTS
- Dystrophin deficiency—demonstrated immunocytochemically or by Western blot analysis; diagnostic
- Serologic testing—may be warranted to rule out infectious and immune-mediated causes

IMAGING
N/A

DIAGNOSTIC PROCEDURES
Electromyography—shows complex repetitive discharges

PATHOLOGIC FINDINGS
Histologic examination of muscle—muscle fiber necrosis and regeneration; myofiber mineralization (may be dramatic); myofiber hypertrophy (may be variation in myofiber size or fibrosis)

 TREATMENT

None proven effective

153

HEREDITARY X-LINKED MUSCULAR DYSTROPHY

 MEDICATIONS

DRUG(S)
Glucocorticosteriods—may provide some improvement; reason unknown

CONTRAINDICATIONS/POSSIBLE INTERACTIONS
None

 FOLLOW-UP

PATIENT MONITORING
Monitor periodically for aspiration pneumonia or cardiomyopathy.

PREVENTION/AVOIDANCE
- Discourage breeding of affected animals.
- Do not repeat dam–sire breedings that result in affected offspring.

POSSIBLE COMPLICATIONS
Aspiration pneumonia or cardiomyopathy may be life threatening.

EXPECTED COURSE AND PROGNOSIS
- Overall prognosis—guarded to poor as no effective palliative treatment
- Golden retrievers—signs tend to stabilize at 6 months.
- Other dog breeds and cats—progression variable

 MISCELLANEOUS

ASSOCIATED CONDITIONS
N/A

AGE-RELATED FACTORS
N/A

ZOONOTIC POTENTIAL
N/A

PREGNANCY
N/A

154

Suggested Reading

Kornegay JN. The X-linked muscular dystrophies. In: Kirk RW, Bonagura JD, eds. Current veterinary therapy XI. Philadelphia: Saunders, 1992:1042–1047.

Author: Georgina Child
Consulting Editor: Peter K. Shires

Myopathy, Noninflammatory– Metabolic

 BASICS

DEFINITION
- Myopathy associated with disorders of glycogen metabolism, lipid metabolism, or oxidative phosphorylation and mitochondrial metabolism
- Currently poorly characterized in veterinary medicine

PATHOPHYSIOLOGY
- Usually associated with inherited or acquired enzyme defects involving major metabolic pathways
- May result in storage of the abnormal metabolic byproduct or morphologic abnormalities of mitochondria

SYSTEMS AFFECTED
- Neuromuscular—dependence on oxidative metabolism for energy
- Nervous—dependence on glycolytic and oxidative metabolism for energy
- Cardiovascular—dependence on oxidative metabolism for energy
- Hemic/Lymphatic/Immune—RBCs depend on glycolytic metabolism.
- Storage products in other organs—liver; spleen

GENETICS
Undetermined

INCIDENCE/PREVALENCE
Rare, except lipid-storage myopathies

GEOGRAPHIC DISTRIBUTION
Unknown; probably worldwide

SIGNALMENT

Species
Dogs and cats

MYOPATHY, NONINFLAMMATORY—METABOLIC

Breed Predilections
- Inherited muscle phosphofructokinase deficiency—English springer spaniels, American cocker spaniels
- Acid maltase deficiency—Laplands
- Debranching enzyme deficiency—German shepherds
- Mitochondrial myopathy—clumber spaniels, Sussex spaniels, Old English sheepdogs

Mean Age and Range
- Inherited metabolic defects—2–3 months
- Acquired metabolic defects—adults

Predominant Sex
None found

SIGNS

General Comments
Very few of these conditions have been adequately described.

Historical Findings
- Muscular weakness
- Exercise intolerance
- Cramping
- Collapse
- Regurgitation and/or dysphagia
- Esophageal and/or pharyngeal abnormalities
- Dark urine; myoglobinuria; hemoglobinuria
- Encephalopathy
- Vomiting

Physical Examination Findings
- Exercise-related weakness, stiffness, and/or cramping
- Abnormal neurologic examination—disorientation; stupor; coma
- Abdominal distention—storage product accumulation in liver
- May appear normal, with fluctuating clinical signs

CAUSES
- Inborn error of metabolism
- Acquired metabolic defect
- Viral infections

157

- Drug induced
- Environmental factors

RISK FACTORS
- Inherited disorders
- Appropriate genetic background
- Others unknown

 DIAGNOSIS

DIFFERENTIAL DIAGNOSIS
- Inflammatory myopathies—differentiated by muscle biopsy
- Other noninflammatory myopathies—differentiated by muscle biopsy
- Other metabolic encephalopathies—differentiated by laboratory evaluation

CBC/BIOCHEMISTRY/URINALYSIS
- Plasma lactate levels—elevated resting or postexcercise with disorders of fatty acid oxidation or oxidative phosphorylation; no elevation with glycolytic disorders
- Serum creatine kinase levels—may be elevated with exercise and normal at rest; may be persistently elevated
- Hypoglycemia—may occur with some glycolytic and oxidative disorders
- Hyperammonemia—may occur with urea cycle defects

OTHER LABORATORY TESTS
- Quantitation of plasma amino acids—abnormal accumulations
- Quantitation of urine organic acids—demonstrate abnormal organic acid production
- Quantitation of plasma, urine, and muscle carnitine—may be low with primary or secondary disorders of carnitine; low with primary organic acidurias
- Specific enzyme assays—depend on suspected metabolic defect
- Fibroblast cultures—study metabolic defect

IMAGING
MRI—evaluate the CNS; reveals abnormalities in humans

MYOPATHY, NONINFLAMMATORY–METABOLIC

DIAGNOSTIC PROCEDURES
- Light microscopy—fresh frozen muscle sections; demonstrates storage products (glycogen, lipid) or abnormal mitochondria
- Electron microscopy of muscle reveals abnormal mitochondria, paracrystalline inclusions, and glycogen or lipid accumulation.
- Cardiovascular system evaluation—may have concurrent cardiomyopathy
- Other organ biopsies—with organomegaly

PATHOLOGIC FINDINGS
- Triglyceride droplets in muscle—lipid storage myopathy
- Ragged-red fibers in muscle—mitochondrial myopathy
- Glycogen deposition in muscle—glycogen storage disorder

 TREATMENT

APPROPRIATE HEALTH CARE
- Inpatient—may required intensive care for severe encephalopathy, seizures, lactic acidemia, hypoglycemia, or hyperammonemia
- Outpatient—clinical signs related only to neuromuscular system

NURSING CARE
Depends on type and severity of disorder

ACTIVITY
Exercise restriction—with muscle weakness, stiffness, or exercise-induced collapse

DIET
- Avoid prolonged periods of fasting.
- Restrictions—depend on underlying defect
- Vitamin and co-factor therapy—determined by underlying defect

CLIENT EDUCATION
- Warn client that most inherited metabolic defects cannot be cured, although some can be treated.
- Advise against breeding affected individuals.

SURGICAL CONSIDERATIONS
N/A

 MEDICATIONS

DRUG(S) OF CHOICE
- Depend on the abnormality and clinical signs
- Lipid storage myopathies—L-carnitine (50 mg/kg PO q12h); riboflavin (50–100 mg PO q24h); coenzyme Q_{10} (1 mg/kg PO q24h)
- Mitochondrial myopathies—may benefit from therapy similar to that listed for lipid storage myopathies

CONTRAINDICATIONS
None known

PRECAUTIONS
Avoid fasting and strenuous exercise if they precipitate clinical signs.

POSSIBLE INTERACTIONS
N/A

ALTERNATIVE DRUG(S)
N/A

 FOLLOW-UP

PATIENT MONITORING
- Lipid storage myopathies—return of muscle strength; elimination of muscle pain
- Elevated serum creatine kinase—should return to normal

PREVENTION/AVOIDANCE
N/A

POSSIBLE COMPLICATIONS
Severe neurologic impairment

EXPECTED COURSE AND PROGNOSIS
- Untreatable disorder—poor prognosis
- Lipid storage myopathies—good prognosis if no underlying organic acidemia

MISCELLANEOUS

ASSOCIATED CONDITIONS
- Iatrogenic and naturally occurring Cushing syndrome
- Lipid storage myopathies—found in some dogs
- Hemolytic anemia—due to underlying metabolic defect

AGE-RELATED FACTORS
- Inborn errors—usually found in young dogs
- Acquired defects—found in adult dogs

ZOONOTIC POTENTIAL
N/A

PREGNANCY
Unknown

SYNONYMS
- Lipid storage myopathies
- Mitochondrial myopathies
- Glycogen storage disorders
- Cori disease—glycogenosis type III
- Phosphofructokinase deficiency—glycogenosis type VII
- Acid maltase deficiency—glycogenosis type II)

ABBREVIATIONS
- CNS = central nervous system
- MRI = magnetic resonance imaging
- RBC = red blood cell

Suggested Reading
Fyfe JC. Molecular diagnosis of inherited neuromuscular disease. Vet Clin North Am 2002;31:287–300.

LeCouteur RA, Dow SW, Sisson AF. Metabolic and endocrine myopathies of dogs and cats. Semin Vet Med Surg Small Anim 1989;4:146–155.

Platt SR. Neuromuscular complications in endocrine and metabolic disorders. Vet Clin North Am 2002;31:125–146.

Shelton GD, Gardinet GH III. Pathophysiologic basis of canine muscle disorders. J Vet Intern Med 1987;1:36–44.

Shelton GD. Canine lipid storage myopathies. In: Bonagura JD, Kirk RW, eds. Current veterinary therapy XII. Philadelphia: Saunders, 1995;1161–1163.

Shelton GD, Engvall E. Muscular dystrophies and other inherited myopathies. Vet Clin North Am 2002;31: 103–124.

Author: G. Diane Shelton
Consulting Editor: Peter K. Shires

Osteochondrodysplasia

 BASICS

OVERVIEW
- A growth and developmental abnormality of cartilage and bone; encompasses many disorders involving bone growth
- Results from delayed endochondral ossification
- Skeletal defects—usually involve the appendicular skeleton; specifically the metaphyseal growth plates
- Achondroplasia—failure of cartilage growth; characterized by a proportionate short-limbed dysplasia; evident soon after birth
- Hypochondrodysplasia—less severe form of achondrodysplasia
- Characteristic breeds—result of selection of certain desirable traits
- Affects musculoskeletal and ophthalmic systems

SIGNALMENT
- Achondroplastic breeds—bulldogs; Boston terriers; pugs; Pekingese; Japanese spaniels; shih tzus
- Hypochondroplastic breeds—dachshunds; basset hounds; beagles; Welsh corgis; dandie Dinmont terriers; Scottish terriers; Skye terriers
- Reported nonselected chondrodysplastic abnormalities—Alaskan malamutes; Samoyeds; Labrador retrievers; English pointers; Norwegian elkhounds; Great Pyrenees; cocker spaniels; Scottish terriers; Scottish deerhounds
- Ocular-skeletal dysplasia—diagnosed in Labrador retrievers and Samoyeds

SIGNS

Historical Findings
- Obvious skeletal deformities
- Retarded growth

OSTEOCHONDRODYSPLASIA

Physical Examination Findings
- Usually affects the appendicular skeleton; may affect axial skeleton
- Long bones—appear shorter than normal; often bowed
- Major joints (elbow, stifle, carpus, tarsus)—appear enlarged
- Radius and ulna—often severely affected owing to asynchronous growth
- Lateral bowing of the forelimbs
- Enlarged carpal joints
- Valgus deformity of the paws
- Shortened maxilla—relative mandibular prognathism
- Spinal deviations—due to hemivertebrae
- Retina—dysplasia; partial to complete detachment

CAUSES & RISK FACTORS
- Achondrodysplastic and hypochondrodysplastic breeds—autosomal dominant trait
- Nonselected chondrodysplastic breeds—simple autosomal recessive or polygenic trait
- Littermates often affected

DIAGNOSIS

DIFFERENTIAL DIAGNOSIS
Premature closure of the ulnar or radial physes—history of trauma; no other bones affected; unilateral or bilateral abnormalities

CBC/BIOCHEMISTRY/URINALYSIS
N/A

OTHER LABORATORY TESTS
N/A

IMAGING
- Radiography of affected limbs—irregular flattening of the metaphysis; widening of the physeal line; retained endochondral cores; irregularities in ossification of the affected long bone; degenerative joint disease and joint

laxity owing to abnormal stress and weight bearing on
the limbs
• Radiography of the spine—hemivertebrae; wedge-
shaped vertebrae

DIAGNOSTIC PROCEDURES
Bone biopsy of growth plate—definitive diagnosis

PATHOLOGIC FINDINGS
Histologic findings: disorganization of the proliferative zone,
abnormalities within the hypertrophic zone, abnormal
formation of the primary and secondary spongiosa

 TREATMENT

• Achondrodysplasia—considered a normal abnormality in
some (chondrodystrophic) breeds
• Surgery—usually of little benefit for nonselected
chondrodysplasia
• Corrective osteotomy to realign limb(s) or joint(s)—may
have limited benefit

 MEDICATIONS

DRUG(S)
• Analgesics and antiinflammatory agents—palliative use
warranted; may try buffered or enteric-coated aspirin
(10–25 mg/kg PO q8h–12h), carprofen (2.2 mg/kg PO
q12h), etodolac (10–15 mg/kg PO q24h), phenylbutazone (3–7 mg/kg PO q8h, total dose < 800 mg/day),
meclofenamic acid (0.5 mg/kg PO q12h), or piroxicam
(0.3 mg/kg PO q24h for 3 days; then every other day)
• Chondroprotective agents—polysulfated glycosaminoglycans, glucosamine, and chondroitin sulfate; may
have limited benefit in preventing articular cartilage
changes

CONTRAINDICATIONS/POSSIBLE INTERACTIONS
N/A

FOLLOW-UP

PREVENTION/AVOIDANCE
- Do not repeat dam–sire breedings that resulted in affected offspring.
- Discourage breeding affected animals.

POSSIBLE COMPLICATIONS
Intra-articular and periarticular joint structures—degenerate owing to abnormal conformation of the appendicular skeleton; leads to altered biomechanics; results in poor quality of life

EXPECTED COURSE AND PROGNOSIS
Depend on severity

 MISCELLANEOUS

SYNONYMS
Dwarfism

Suggested Reading
Sande RD, Bingel SA. Animal models of dwarfism. Vet Clin North Am Small Anim Pract 1982;13:71.

Author: Peter D. Schwarz
Consulting Editor: Peter K. Shires

Osteochondrosis

BASICS

DEFINITION
A pathologic process in growing cartilage, primarily characterized by a disturbance of endochondral ossification that leads to excessive retention of cartilage

PATHOPHYSIOLOGY
- Cells of the immature articular joint cartilage and growth plates do not differentiate normally.
- The process of endochondral ossification is retarded, but the cartilage continues to grow, resulting in abnormally thick regions that are less resistant to mechanical stress.
- Bilateral disease common
- Most commonly affected joints—shoulder (caudocentral humeral head); elbow (medial aspect humeral condyle); stifle (femoral condyle: lateral more often than medial); hock (ridge of the talus: medial more common than lateral)
- Other reported locations—femoral head; dorsal rim of the acetabulum; glenoid cavity (scapula); patella; distal radius; medial malleolus; cranial end plate of the sacrum; vertebral articular facets; cervical vertebrae

Immature Joint Cartilage
- Nutrition maintained by diffusion of nutrients from the synovial fluid
- Thickened cartilage results in impaired metabolism, leading to degeneration and necrosis of the poorly supplied cells
- Fissure within the thickened cartilage—may result from mechanical stress; eventually leads to the formation of a cartilage flap, or OCD; may cause lameness
- Lameness (pain)—becomes evident once synovial fluid establishes contact with subchondral bone; affected by cartilage breakdown products released into the synovial fluid; inflammation

167

OSTEOCHONDROSIS

Retention of Cartilage in Growth Plates
- Usually does not lead to necrosis, probably owing to nutrition provided by vessels within the cartilage
- May lead to slippage and asymmetric growth; most marked in the distal ulnar physis

SYSTEMS AFFECTED
Musculoskeletal

GENETICS
- Polygenetic transmission—expression determined by an interaction of genetic and environmental factors
- Heritability index—depends on breed; 0.25–0.45

INCIDENCE/PREVALENCE
Frequent and serious problem in many dog breeds

GEOGRAPHIC DISTRIBUTION
N/A

SIGNALMENT

Species
- Dogs
- Demonstrated clinically—horses; pigs; broiler chickens; turkeys; humans

Breed Predilections
Large and giant breeds—great Danes, Labrador retrievers, Newfoundlands, rottweilers, Bernese mountain dogs, English setters, Old English sheepdogs

Mean Age and Range
- Onset of clinical signs—typically 4–8 months
- Diagnosis—generally 4–18 months
- Symptoms of secondary DJD—any age

Predominant Sex
- Shoulder—males (2:1)
- Elbow, stifle, and hock—none

SIGNS

General Comments
Depend on the affected joint(s) and concurrent DJD

Historical Findings

Lameness—most common; sudden or insidious in onset; one or more limbs; becomes worse after exercise; duration of several weeks to months; slight, moderate, or severe; patient may support little weight on the affected limb.

Physical Examination Findings

- Pain—usually elicited on palpation by flexing, extending, or rotating the involved joint
- Generally a weight-bearing lameness
- Joint effusion with capsular distention—common with OCD of elbow, stifle, and hock
- Muscle atrophy—consistent finding with chronic lameness
- Hock OCD—hyperextension of the tarsocrural joint

CAUSES

- Developmental
- Nutritional

RISK FACTORS

- Diet containing three times the recommended calcium levels
- Rapid growth and weight gain

 DIAGNOSIS

DIFFERENTIAL DIAGNOSIS

- Intraarticular (osteochondral) fractures
- Elbow dysplasia
- Panosteitis

CBC/BIOCHEMISTRY/URINALYSIS

N/A

OTHER LABORATORY TESTS

N/A

IMAGING

Radiography

- Standard craniocaudal and mediolateral views—necessary for all involved joints
- Appears as flattening of the subchondral bone or as a subchondral lucency

OSTEOCHONDROSIS

- Cannot be differentiated from OCD
- Sclerosis of the underlying bone—common in chronic OCD lesions; may see flap if it is calcified
- Calcified bodies within the joint (joint mice)—indicate dislodged cartilage flap
- Contralateral joint—comparison; check for involvement
- Oblique views—may improve visualization, especially for hock, elbow, and shoulder lesions
- Skyline views of the talar ridges of the hock joint—help identify medial and lateral lesions

CT and MRI
- Useful for visualizing extent of subchondral lesions
- Not reliable for detecting a loose cartilage flap

Positive Contrast Arthrography
Useful for differentiating from OCD of the shoulder

DIAGNOSTIC PROCEDURES
- Joint tap and analysis of synovial fluid—confirms involvement; should note straw-colored fluid with normal to decreased viscosity; from cytology, should note >10,000 nucleated cells/μL (> 90% should be mononuclear cells)
- Arthroscopy—minimally invasive; excellent method for differentiating from OCD and for corrective treatment

PATHOLOGIC FINDINGS
- Articular cartilage—initially may appear yellowish
- Retention of articular cartilage extending into subchondral bone surrounded by increased amount of trabecular bone
- Clefts between the underlying trabecular bone and the degenerated and necrotic deep layer of the overlying thickened (retained) cartilage

 TREATMENT

APPROPRIATE HEALTH CARE
Not treatable

NURSING CARE
- Cryotherapy (ice packing) of affected joint—immediately postsurgery; 15–20 min three times a day for 3–5 days

- Range-of-motion exercises—initiated as soon as patient can tolerate

ACTIVITY
- Restricted
- Avoid hard concussive activities (e.g., running on concrete).

DIET
- Weight control—important for decreasing load and, therefore, the stress on the affected joint(s)

CLIENT EDUCATION
- Discuss the heritability of the disease.
- Warn client that DJD may develop.
- Discuss the influence of excessive intake of nutrients that promote rapid growth.

SURGICAL CONSIDERATIONS
- Nonsurgical condition
- May progress to OCD as the patient grows
- Arthrotomy or arthroscopy—indicated for most OCD patients
- Shoulder—indicated for all OCD lesions; exploratory procedure indicated for pain and lameness with radiographic evidence of osteochondrosis
- Elbow—indicated for all OCD lesions; indicated to assess for other conditions (see Elbow Dysplasia)
- Stifle—controversial; patients develop DJD even with procedure; arthroscopy may improve the recovery rate and long-term function
- Hock—remove osteochondral flap; controversial; all patients develop severe DJD even with procedure; attempt to reattach the flap to the underlying subchondral bone, if warranted.

 MEDICATIONS

DRUG(S) OF CHOICE
Antiinflammatory drugs (NSAIDs) and analgesics—may be used to symptomatically treat associated DJD; do not promote healing of the cartilage flap (thus surgery is still indicated)

OSTEOCHONDROSIS

CONTRAINDICATIONS
Avoid corticosteroids owing to potential side effects and articular cartilage damage associated with long-term use.

PRECAUTIONS
NSAIDs—gastrointestinal irritation may preclude their use.

POSSIBLE INTERACTIONS
N/A

ALTERNATIVE DRUG(S)
Chondroprotective drugs (e.g., polysulfated glycosaminogly-cans, glucosamine, and chondroitin sulfate)—may help limit cartilage damage and degeneration; may help alleviate pain and inflammation

 FOLLOW-UP

PATIENT MONITORING
- Periodic monitoring until patient is skeletally mature—recommended to assess progression to an OCD lesion
- Postsurgery—limit activity for 4–6 weeks; encourage early, active movement of the affected joint(s).
- Yearly examinations—recommended to assess progression of DJD

PREVENTION/AVOIDANCE
- Discourage breeding of patients.
- Do not repeat dam–sire breedings that resulted in affected offspring.
- Restricted weight gain and growth in young dogs—may decrease incidence

POSSIBLE COMPLICATIONS
N/A

EXPECTED COURSE AND PROGNOSIS
- Shoulder—good to excellent prognosis for return to full function; minimal osteoarthritis development
- Elbow, stifle, and hock—fair to guarded prognosis; depends on size of lesion (most important), DJD, and age at diagnosis and treatment; progressive osteoarthritis development, even after surgery

MISCELLANEOUS

ASSOCIATED CONDITIONS
N/A

AGE-RELATED FACTORS
N/A

ZOONOTIC POTENTIAL
N/A

PREGNANCY
N/A

SEE ALSO
Elbow Dysplasia

ABBREVIATIONS
- CT = computed tomography
- DJD = degenerative joint disease
- MRI = magnetic resonance imaging
- NSAID = nonsteroidal antiinflammatory drug
- OCD = osteochondritis dissecans

Suggested Reading

Fox SM, Walker AM. The etiopathogenesis of osteochondrosis. Vet Med 1993;88:116–122.

Olsson SE. Lameness in the dog: a review of lesion causing osteoarthrosis of the shoulder, elbow, hip, stifle and hock joints. Proceedings of the American Animal Hospital Association, 1975;42:363–370.

Olsson SE. Osteochondritis dissecans in dogs: a study of pathogenesis, clinical signs, pathologic changes, natural course and sequelae [Abstract]. J Am Vet Radiol Soc 1973;14:4.

Author: Peter D. Schwarz
Consulting Editor: Peter K. Shires

Osteomyelitis

BASICS

DEFINITION
An acute or chronic inflammation of bone and the associated soft tissue elements of marrow, endosteum, periosteum and vascular channels that is usually caused by bacteria and rarely by fungi and other microorganisms

PATHOPHYSIOLOGY
- Hematogenously disseminated microorganisms—may localize in metaphyseal bone of young animals and vertebrae of adults; cause osteomyelitis when tissue defense mechanisms have been compromised
- Direct inoculation of bone with pathogenic bacteria—may not initiate infection unless there is concurrent tissue injury, bone necrosis, sequestration, fracture instability, altered tissue defenses, foreign material, or surgical implants
- Once bone infection is established, bacteria may persist by adhering to implants and sequestra.
- Biofilm—made up of slime produced by staphylococci and other bacteria together with host-derived proteins, cellular debris, and carbohydrate; enshrouds bacterial colonies; provides protection from antimicrobial drugs and host defenses; induces some bacteria to transform to more virulent strains that are more resistant to antimicrobial drugs
- Fracture instability exacerbates infection; resorption of bone owing to infection and instability causes widening of the fracture gap and implant loosening, contributing to persistence of infection.

SYSTEMS AFFECTED
Musculoskeletal

GENETICS
Breeds with heritable immunodeficiency or hematogenous diseases

INCIDENCE/PREVALENCE
- Prevalence after open reduction and internal fixation of closed fractures not uncommon (probably similar incidence as diskospondylitis)
- Prevalence after trauma and open fracture—unknown; relatively common
- Hematogenous disease in young dogs—uncommon
- Diskospondylitis in adult dogs and cats and fungal disease—not uncommon

GEOGRAPHIC DISTRIBUTION
- Actinomycosis—grass awns usually cause soft tissue infections, not osteomyelitis; with osteomyelitis, likely a soil contaminant: California, Florida, UK, and Australia
- Blastomycosis—central and eastern regions of the U.S: Great Lakes region and the Mississippi and Ohio River valleys
- Coccidioidomycosis—southwestern U.S., Mexico, and Central and South America
- Histoplasmosis—Ohio, Missouri, and Mississippi River valleys and tributaries

SIGNALMENT

Species
Dogs and cats

Breed Predilections
Breeds with immunodeficiency and hematogenous diseases

Mean Age and Range
Hematogenous metaphyseal infection—young dogs

Predominant Sex
Male dogs—for post-traumatic infection; blastomycosis

SIGNS

General Comments
- Acute postoperative wound infections after orthopedic surgery—may be indistinguish-able from acute condition; may progress to chronic disease
- Most patients have chronic disease at time of examination and diagnosis.

OSTEOMYELITIS

Historical Findings
- Episodes of lameness
- Draining tracts
- Persistent ulcers
- Previous trauma
- Fracture or surgery—post-traumatic disease
- Affected vertebrae or intervertebral disks (dogs)—may note hind limb weakness and difficulty in rising
- Travel to regions endemic for mycotic infections—fungal infection

Physical Examination Findings
- Acute hematogenous disease (dogs)—sudden onset of systemic illness; pyrexia; lethargy; limb pain; local signs of acute inflammation
- Chronic condition—usually associated with chronic draining tracts, nonhealing ulcers, pain, secondary muscle atrophy, and joint stiffness
- Unhealed fractures with concurrent infection—may note instability, crepitus, and limb deformity
- Fungal infections—may see limb swelling, lameness, and intermittently draining tracts
- Bone infections of the spine—may cause pain and neurologic deficits (e.g., paresis and paralysis)

CAUSES
- Open fracture
- Traumatic injury
- Open reduction and internal fixation of closed fracture
- Elective orthopedic surgery
- Prosthetic joint implant
- Gunshot wound
- Penetrating foreign body
- Bite and claw wounds
- Extension to bone of soft tissue infection—periodontitis; rhinitis; otitis media; paronychia
- Hematogenous infection
- Staphylococci—cause approximately 50% of bone infections; often monomicrobial infections
- Polymicrobial infection—common; may contain mixtures of aerobic gram-negative bacteria; anaerobic cultures

should be submitted with potential isolates including: *Actinomyces, Clostridium, Peptostreptococcus, Bacteroides,* and *Fusobacterium*
- Fungal infection—*Coccidioides immitis; Blastomyces dermatitidis; Histoplasma capsulatum; Cryptococcus neoformans; Aspergillus*

RISK FACTORS
- Open fracture and bone contamination
- Soft tissue trauma
- Bite and claw wounds
- Migrating foreign body
- Orthopedic surgery
- Prosthetic orthopedic implant
- Cortical bone allograft
- Immunodeficiency

 DIAGNOSIS

DIFFERENTIAL DIAGNOSIS
- Neoplasia
- Bone cysts
- Delayed fracture union as a result of instability
- Hypertrophic osteodystrophy
- Secondary hypertrophic osteopathy
- Medullary bone infarction

CBC/BIOCHEMISTRY/URINALYSIS
Hemogram—inflammatory left shift usually evident only with acute disease

OTHER LABORATORY TESTS
Serology—confirms some fungal infections

IMAGING

Radiology
- Acute disease—bone architecture normal; see only soft tissue swelling
- Chronic disease—sequestra (avascular segment of cortical bone); reactive periosteal new bone; involucrum formation (reactive tissue surrounding sequestrum); bone resorption

OSTEOMYELITIS

- Bone resorption—widening of fracture gaps; cortical thinning; generalized osteopenia; implant loosening
- Contrast films—may help delineate sinuses and radiolucent foreign bodies; inject water-soluble contrast media through a Foley catheter into the sinuses.

Other
- Ultrasonography—localize large accumulations of fluid; guide fluid sampling by needle aspiration
- Scintigraphy—^{99m}Tc-labeled methylene diphosphonate; highly sensitive for detecting increased vascularity of bone; not specific for osteomyelitis

DIAGNOSTIC PROCEDURES
- Fluid aspirates or Jamshidi-needle tissue biopsies—collected from focus of infection by sterile techniques; cultured aerobically and anaerobically; identify microorganisms; determine in vitro antimicrobial drug susceptibility
- Open surgical biopsy—indicated when needle aspirates are negative or when débridement is necessary for treatment; culture samples of necrotic tissue, sequestra, implants, and foreign material; histopathologic examination for suspected fungal infection and to rule-out neoplasia
- Fluid and tissue samples for anaerobic culture—immediately place into appropriate medium (e.g., reduced Cary-Blair anaerobic transport medium).
- Purulent fluid from draining tracts—culture may be misleading; tracts are colonized by skin organisms and gram-negative bacteria; cultures are often polymicrobic.
- Blood cultures—may be positive with acute disease or chronic disease with septicemia.

PATHOLOGIC FINDINGS
- Bone sequestration—virtually diagnostic
- Inflammation and necrosis of bone and the adjacent tissues—pyogenic bacteria
- Cytologic or histopathologic examination of smears or sections—usually leads to diagnosis of fungal infection; special fungal stains (methenamine silver; PAS) for microorganism identification

TREATMENT

APPROPRIATE HEALTH CARE
- Inpatient—surgical débridement, drainage, culturing, irrigation, and wound management until infection begins to resolve; infected fractures (surgical stabilization)
- Outpatient—long-term oral antimicrobial drug therapy

NURSING CARE
- Depends on severity, location, and degree of associated soft tissue injury
- Take care to prevent nosocomial infections by pathogen contamination to other patients in the hospital.

ACTIVITY
Restricted—with any danger of a pathologic fracture developing; with an unhealed fracture

DIET
No restriction

CLIENT EDUCATION
- Warn the client about the expense of treatment, the likelihood of recurrence, the problems with sequestration, the need for repeated surgical intervention, and the long duration of therapy.
- Discuss the prognosis.

SURGICAL CONSIDERATIONS
- Chronic disease—surgical débridement; removal of sequestrum; establishment of drainage
- Infected stable fracture—leave pre-existing internal fixation implants in place during healing.
- Infected unstable fracture—remove implants; stabilize with external or internal skeletal fixation.
- Bone deficits—graft with autologous cancellous bone either acutely or after infection has abated and granulation tissue has formed in the wound.
- Large segmental deficits in long bones—bridge by Ilizarov technique or other bone segment transport.
- Localized chronic infection—may be amenable to resolution by amputation (tail, digit, limb) or en bloc resection

(sternum, thoracic wall, mandible, maxilla) and primary wound closure
- Remove all implants after the fracture has healed; bacteria harbored by implant biofilm may lead to recurrence or be a pathogenic factor for fracture-associated sarcoma.

 MEDICATIONS

DRUG(S) OF CHOICE
- Antimicrobial drugs—depend on in vitro determination of susceptibility of microorganisms; also consider possible toxicity, frequency and route of administration, and expense; most penetrate normal and infected bone well; must be given for 4–8 weeks
- Staphylococci (dogs)—usually *S. intermedius,* which are resistant to penicillin because of b-lactamase production; highly susceptible to cloxacillin, amoxicillin-clavulanate, cefazolin, and clindamycin
- Anaerobes—more are sensitive to metronidazole and clindamycin.
- Aminoglycosides and quinolones (ciprofloxacin and enrofloxacin)—effective against gram-negative aerobic bacteria
- Quinolones—may give orally; not nephrotoxic; to protect against resistance, use only for infections caused by gram-negative organisms or *Pseudomonas* that are resistant to other oral antimicrobial drugs.
- Chronic disease—continuous local delivery of antimicrobial drugs by antibiotic-impregnated methylmethacrylate beads
- Itraconazole—5–10 mg/kg PO q24h; given continuously, may control disseminated aspergillosis for up to 2 years

CONTRAINDICATIONS
Quinolones—do not give to young patients; experimentally induce articular cartilage lesions in immature dogs

PRECAUTIONS
Aminoglycosides—may cause nephrotoxicity, especially in dehydrated patients and with electrolyte losses or pre-existing renal disease

POSSIBLE INTERACTIONS
N/A

ALTERNATIVE DRUG(S)
Identify other antimicrobial drugs by repeating cultures and susceptibility determination if the infection becomes unresponsive to the initial agent.

 FOLLOW-UP

PATIENT MONITORING
- Radiography—every 4–6 weeks; determine bone healing
- Reculture bone—suspected persistent infection

PREVENTION/AVOIDANCE
N/A

POSSIBLE COMPLICATIONS
- Recurrence
- Chronic disease—may result in limb deformity, impaired function, fracture disease, or neurologic deficits
- Malignant neoplasia—rare sequela to chronic infection of fractures repaired by internal fixation

EXPECTED COURSE AND PROGNOSIS
- Acute infection and chronic bacterial diskospondylitis—may be cured by 4–8 weeks of antimicrobial drug therapy if there is limited bone necrosis and no fracture
- Chronic disease—resolution with antimicrobial drug therapy alone unlikely; provide appropriate surgical treatment.
- Recurrence of chronic infection—evident by return of lameness or draining tracts; may occur weeks, months, or years after the last treatment; may require repeated sequestrectomy, débridement, microbiologic culturing, drainage, fracture stabilization, bone grafting, or implant removal

 MISCELLANEOUS

ASSOCIATED CONDITIONS
N/A

OSTEOMYELITIS

AGE-RELATED FACTORS
N/A

ZOONOTIC POTENTIAL
N/A

PREGNANCY
N/A

SYNONYMS
Bone infection

SEE ALSO
- Diskospondylitis

Suggested Reading

Doherty MA, Smith MM. Contamination and infection of fractures resulting from gunshot trauma in dogs: 20 cases (1987–1992). J Am Vet Med Assoc 1995;206(2): 203–205.

Johnson KA. Osteomyelitis. In: Birchard SJ, Sherding RG, eds. Saunders manual of small animal practice. Philadelphia: Saunders, 1994:1091–1095.

Johnson KA. Osteomyelitis in dogs and cats. J Am Vet Med Assoc 1994;205:1882–1887.

Rochat MC. Preventing and treating osteomyelitis. Vet Med 2001;96(a).

Authors: Kenneth A. Johnson and Mark M. Smith
Consulting Editor: Peter K. Shires

Panosteitis

BASICS

DEFINITION
A self-limiting, painful condition affecting one or more of the long bones of young, medium- to large-breed dogs that is characterized clinically by lameness and radiographically by high density of the marrow cavity.

PATHOPHYSIOLOGY
- Cause unknown
- Attempts to isolate microorganisms have failed
- Metabolic, allergic, or endocrine aberrations—without support
- Pain—may be owing to disturbance of endosteal and periosteal elements, vascular congestion, or high intramedullary pressure

SYSTEMS AFFECTED
Musculoskeletal—lameness of variable intensity; may affect a single limb or become a shifting leg lameness

GENETICS
- No proven transmission
- Predominance of German shepherds in the affected population strongly suggests an inheritable basis.

INCIDENCE/PREVALENCE
No reliable estimates; common

GEOGRAPHIC DISTRIBUTION
N/A

SIGNALMENT

Species
Dogs

PANOSTEITIS

Breed Predilections
- German shepherds and German shepherd mixes—most commonly affected
- Medium to large breeds—most commonly affected

Mean Age and Range
- Usually 5–18 months of age
- As young as 2 months and as old as 5 years

Predominant Sex
Male

SIGNS

General Comments
Lameness—if no distinct abnormalities noted on physical examination or radiographs, repeat examinations 4-6 weeks later.

Historical Findings
- No associated trauma
- Lameness—varying intensity; usually involves the fore-limbs initially; may affect the hind limbs; may see shifting leg lameness; may be non–weight bearing
- Severe disease—mild depression; inappetence; weight loss

Physical Examination Findings
- Pain—on deep palpation of the long bones (diaphysis) in an affected limb; distinguishing characteristic; palpate firmly along the entire shaft of each bone while carefully avoiding any pinching of nearby muscle.
- Bones—ulna most commonly affected; may affect radius, humerus, femur, and tibia (in decreasing order of frequency) either concurrently or subsequently
- May note low-grade fever
- May see muscle atrophy

CAUSES
Unknown

RISK FACTORS
Purebred German shepherd or German shepherd mix

DIAGNOSIS

DIFFERENTIAL DIAGNOSIS
- Always consider the diagnosis with lameness in a young German shepherd or German shepherd mix.
- May occur alone or with other juvenile orthopedic diseases
- Osteochondritis dissecans
- Fragmented medial coronoid process
- Un-united anconeal process
- Hip dysplasia
- Fractures and ligamentous injuries from unobserved trauma
- Shifting leg lameness—immune-mediated arthritides; Lyme disease; bacterial endocarditis
- Coccidioidomycosis
- Bacterial osteomyelitis

CBC/BIOCHEMISTRY/URINALYSIS
- Usually normal
- May note eosinophilia early in disease

OTHER LABORATORY TESTS
N/A

IMAGING
- Radiographic densities within the medulla of long bones—characteristic; confirm diagnosis
- Early, middle, and late radiographic lesions
- Early—trabecular pattern of the ends of the diaphysis becomes more prominent; may appear blurred; may see granular opacities
- Middle—patchy sclerotic opacities first around the nutrient foramen and later throughout the diaphysis; widened cortex; thickened periosteum with increased opacity
- Late—during resolution, diminished overall opacity of the medullary canal (toward normal); a coarse trabecular pattern and some granular opacity may remain; may be a period in which the medullary canal becomes more lucent than normal

PANOSTEITIS

DIAGNOSTIC PROCEDURES
Bone biopsy—occasionally indicated to rule out neoplasia and bacterial or fungal infections that have similar radiographic appearances

PATHOLOGIC FINDINGS
- Biopsy or necropsy—rarely performed because of excellent prognosis for recovery
- No gross pathologic lesions
- Degeneration of the marrow adipocytes surrounding the nutrient foramen followed by proliferation of vascular stromal cells within the marrow sinusoids
- Osteoid formation and endosteal new bone formation—progress proximally and distally
- Vascular congestion—may accompany the proliferation of new bone, secondarily stimulating endosteal and periosteal reaction
- Remodeling of the endosteum—occurs during resolution; reestablishes normal endosteal and marrow architecture

TREATMENT

APPROPRIATE HEALTH CARE
Outpatient

NURSING CARE
Maintenance and replacement fluid therapy—occasionally owing to prolonged periods of inappetence and pyrexia

ACTIVITY
- Limited—not shown to hasten recovery; lessens pain
- Moderate to severe disease—pain may cause self-limited movement leading to muscle atrophy.

DIET
N/A

CLIENT EDUCATION
- Warn client that patient may develop other juvenile orthopedic diseases.
- Inform client that signs of pain and lameness may last for several weeks.

- Warn client that recurrence of clinical signs is common up to 2 years of age.

SURGICAL CONSIDERATIONS
N/A

 MEDICATIONS

DRUG(S) OF CHOICE

NSAIDs
- Minimize pain; decrease inflammation
- Symptomatic therapy has no bearing on the duration of the disease.
- May try buffered or enteric-coated aspirin (10–25 mg/kg PO q8h or q12h), carprofen (2.2 mg/kg PO q12h), etodolac (10–15 mg/kg PO q24h), phenylbutazone (3–7 mg/kg PO q8h, total dose < 800 mg/day), meclofenamic acid (0.5 mg/kg PO q12h), or piroxicam (0.3 mg/kg PO q24h for 3 days, then q48h)

Glucocorticoids
- May give antiinflammatory dosage—prednisone (0.1–0.5 mg/kg PO)
- Potential side affects well documented
- Goal for chronic use—low-dose and alternate-day therapy

CONTRAINDICATIONS
NSAIDs—gastrointestinal upset may preclude use.

PRECAUTIONS
- NSAIDs—most cause some degree of gastric ulceration.
- Acetaminophen—unsuitable; potential for toxicity

POSSIBLE INTERACTIONS
NSAIDs—do not use in conjunction with glucocorticoids; risk of gastrointestinal tract ulceration

ALTERNATIVE DRUG(S)
N/A

PANOSTEITIS

 FOLLOW-UP

PATIENT MONITORING
Recheck lameness every 2–4 weeks to detect more serious concurrent orthopedic problems.

PREVENTION/AVOIDANCE
N/A

POSSIBLE COMPLICATIONS
N/A

EXPECTED COURSE AND PROGNOSIS
- Self-limiting disease
- Treatment—symptomatic; appears to have no influence on duration of clinical signs.
- Multiple limb involvement—common
- Lameness—typically lasts from a few days to several weeks; may persist for months

 MISCELLANEOUS

ASSOCIATED CONDITIONS
N/A

AGE-RELATED FACTORS
Typically affects immature and young dogs

ZOONOTIC POTENTIAL
N/A

PREGNANCY
Females reported to be more susceptible to panosteitis during estrus; no proven relationship to reproductive hormones or pregnancy

SYNONYMS
- Enostosis
- Fibrous osteodystrophy
- Juvenile osteomyelitis
- Eosinophilic panosteitis

ABBREVIATION

NSAIDs = nonsteroidal antiinflammatory drugs

Suggested Reading

Piermattei DL, Flo GL. Disease conditions in small animals. In: Piermattei DL, Flo GL, eds. Handbook of small animal orthopedics and fracture treatment. 3rd ed. Philadelphia: Saunders, 1997:715–718.

Halliwell WH. Tumorlike lesions of bone. In: Bojrab MJ, ed. Disease mechanisms in small animal surgery. 2nd ed. Philadelphia: Saunders, 1993:932–933.

Manly PA, Romich JA. Miscellaneous orthopedic diseases. In: Slatter DH, ed. Textbook of small animal surgery. 2nd ed. Philadelphia: Saunders, 1993:1984–1987.

Muir P, Dubielzig RR, Johnson KA. Panosteitis. Compend Contin Educ Pract Vet 1996;18:29–33.

Author: Larry Carpenter
Consulting Editor: Peter K. Shires

Patellar Luxation

BASICS

DEFINITION
Medial or lateral displacement of the patella from its normal anatomic position in the femoral trochlea

PATHOPHYSIOLOGY
- May be mild to severe; different degrees of clinical and pathologic changes; classified into grades I–IV
- Common musculoskeletal changes—tibial rotation on its long axis; bowing of the distal and proximal tibia; shallow to absent femoral trochlea; dysplasia of the femoral and tibial epiphysis; displacement of the quadriceps muscle group

SYSTEMS AFFECTED
Musculoskeletal

GENETICS
- Recessive, polygenic, and multifocal inheritances proposed
- Hereditary factor in Devon rex cats

INCIDENCE/PREVALENCE
- One of the most common stifle joint abnormalities in dogs
- Medial—> 75% of cases
- Bilateral involvement—50% of cases
- Uncommon in cats, but may be more common than suspected because most affected cats are not lame

GEOGRAPHIC DISTRIBUTION
N/A

SIGNALMENT

Species
- Predominantly dogs
- Rarely cats

Breed Predilections
- Most common in toy and miniature dog breeds
- Dogs—miniature and toy poodles; Yorkshire terriers; Pomeranians; Pekingese; Chihuahuas; Boston terriers

Mean Age and Range
Clinical signs—may develop soon after birth; generally after 4 months of age

Predominant Sex
Risk for females 1.5 times that for males

SIGNS

General Comments
Depend on grade (severity), amount of degenerative arthritis, chronicity of disease, and occurrence of other stifle joint abnormalities (e.g., cruciate ligament rupture)

Historical Findings
- Persistent abnormal hindlimb carriage and function in neonates and puppies
- Occasional skipping or intermittent hindlimb lameness—worsens in young to mature dogs
- Sudden signs of lameness—owing to minor trauma or worsening DJD in mature animals

Physical Examination Findings
- Grade I—patella can be manually luxated; patella reduces when pressure is released.
- Grade II—patella can be manually luxated or can spontaneously luxate with flexion of the stifle joint; patella remains luxated until it is manually reduced or the patient extends the joint and derotates the tibia in the opposite direction of luxation.
- Grades I and II—patient intermittently carries the affected limb with the stifle joint flexed.
- Grade III—patella remains luxated most of the time but can be manually reduced with the stifle joint in extension; flexion and extension of the stifle joint result in reluxation of the patella.
- Grade IV—patella is permanently luxated and cannot be manually repositioned; may be up to 90° of rotation of

the proximal tibial plateau; shallow or missing femoral trochlea; displacement of quadriceps muscle group in the direction of luxation
- Grades III and IV—crouching, bowlegged (genu varum) or knock-kneed (genu valgum) stance for medial or lateral luxations, respectively; most of the body weight is transferred to the front limbs.
- Pain—may be elicited with chondromalacia of the patella or femoral trochlea

CAUSES
- Congenital
- Traumatic

RISK FACTORS
- Coxa vara—decreased femoral neck–femoral shaft axis; associated with medial luxation
- Coxa valga—increased femoral neck–femoral shaft axis; associated with lateral luxation
- Excessive anteversion—forward inclination of the femoral head and neck

 DIAGNOSIS

DIFFERENTIAL DIAGNOSIS
- Cranial cruciate ligament rupture—distinguished by palpation of cranial drawer motion; concurrent in 15%–20% of cases
- Avulsion fracture of the tibial tubercle—causes laxity of the quadriceps mechanism; results in patellar instability
- Rupture of the patellar tendon—causes proximal displacement of the patella and instability
- Malunion and malalignment of fractures of the femur or tibia—may result in displacement of the quadriceps muscle group
- Craniodorsal hip luxation—often concurrent with grade I luxation owing to laxity of the quadriceps muscle group; laxity spontaneously resolves after reduction of the hip luxation.

CBC/BIOCHEMISTRY/URINALYSIS
N/A

OTHER LABORATORY TESTS
N/A

IMAGING
- Craniocaudal and mediolateral radiographs of the stifle joint—indicated for all grade III and IV luxations; include the joint above (hip) and below (hock) to detect bowing and/or torsion of the femur and tibia.
- Skyline radiographs of the femoral trochlea—help determine its shape (shallow, flattened, or convex)

DIAGNOSTIC PROCEDURES
Arthrocentesis and synovial fluid analysis—slightly increase in mononuclear cells (generally < 2000 cells/mL)

PATHOLOGIC FINDINGS
- Gross—cartilage wear lesions of the patella and femoral trochlea; osteophytes at the joint capsule–bone interface; joint capsule redundancy on the side opposite of luxation; fibrosis and contracture on the side of luxation
- Microscopic—cartilage fibrillation and loss of glycosaminoglycan content; synovitis

 TREATMENT

APPROPRIATE HEALTH CARE
- Outpatient—all grade I and some grade II luxations
- Inpatient (surgery)—most grade II and all grade III and IV luxations

NURSING CARE
- Cryotherapy (ice packing)—initiated immediately after surgery; 15–20 min every 8 hr for 3–5 days
- Range-of-motion exercises of the stifle joint—as soon as tolerated

ACTIVITY
Normal to restricted, depending on severity

DIET
Weight control—important for decreasing the load and, therefore, stress on the stifle joint

193

PATELLAR LUXATION

CLIENT EDUCATION
- Discuss the heritability of the condition.
- Warn client of the possibility of DJD development.
- Inform client of the increased risk of cranial cruciate ligament disease.
- Warn client that the condition could worsen over time (e.g., from grade I to grade II).

SURGICAL CONSIDERATIONS
- Bone deformity (e.g., shallow trochlea or tibial tubercle deviation)—requires surgical bone reconstruction; assumed in all grade II or higher luxations
- Trochleoplasty—arthroplastic procedure; deepen trochlear sulcus
- Trochlear sulcoplasty—curettage technique; remove hyaline cartilage and cancellous bone to deepen the sulcus; fibrocartilage eventually resurfaces the trochlea.
- Recession sulcoplasty—taco shell technique; remove a V-shaped wedge; preserves the hyaline cartilage; after the trochlea is deepened, the osteochondral bone wedge is replaced; creates a new sulcus composed of hyaline cartilage; preferred technique for most patients
- Trochlear chondroplasty—cartilage flap technique; useful only in young patients (< 6 months); create a distally based cartilage flap; remove subchondral bone beneath it; replace flap to line the new sulcus; preserves hyaline cartilage to cover the bottom of the sulcus; fibrocartilage covers the sides.
- Transposition of the tibial tubercle—realign the longitudinal axis of the quadriceps mechanism so that it is centered over the femoral trochlea; osteotomize the tibia tubercle, transpose it opposite the direction of luxation, and stabilize it with pins and a tension band wire.
- Imbrication of the joint capsule and supporting soft tissues on the side opposite the luxation—helps pull the patella over
- Desmotomy or releasing incision—made on the side toward which the patella is luxated
- Patellar and tibial antirotational suture ligaments—reinforce stretched supporting soft tissue structures

- Corrective osteotomy—realigns the longitudinal axis of the hindlimb; generally indicated in only grade III and IV luxations

 MEDICATIONS

DRUG(S) OF CHOICE
NSAIDs—minimize pain; decrease inflammation; may try buffered or enteric-coated aspirin (10–25 mg/kg PO q8–12h), carprofen (2.2 mg/kg PO q12h), etodolac (10–15 mg/kg PO once daily), phenylbutazone (3–7 mg/kg PO q8h, total dose < 800 mg/day), meclofenamic acid (0.5 mg/kg PO q12h), or piroxicam (0.3 mg/kg PO q24h for 3 days, then q48h), or deracoxib (3–4 mg/kg PO q24h for 7 days for postoperative pain) (1–2 mg/kg PO q24h for long-term treatment over 7 days)

CONTRAINDICATIONS
Avoid corticosteroids because of potential side effects and articular cartilage damage associated with long-term use.

PRECAUTIONS
NSAIDs—gastrointestinal irritation may preclude their use.

POSSIBLE INTERACTIONS
N/A

ALTERNATIVE DRUG(S)
Chondroprotective drugs (e.g., polysulfated glycosaminoglycans, glucosamine, and chondroitin sulfate)—may help limit cartilage damage and degeneration

 FOLLOW-UP

PATIENT MONITORING
- Post-trochleoplasty—encourage early, active use of the limb.
- Limit exercise for 4 weeks; prevent jumping.
- Onset of an acute non–weight-bearing lameness—may indicate cranial cruciate ligament disease
- Yearly examinations—to assess progression

PATELLAR LUXATION

PREVENTION/AVOIDANCE
- Discourage breeding of affected animals.
- Do not repeat dam–sire breedings that result in affected offspring.

POSSIBLE COMPLICATIONS
Recurrence after surgical stabilization—reported to be as high as 48%; usually of a lower grade than the original luxation

EXPECTED COURSE AND PROGNOSIS
- With surgical treatment— > 90% of patients are free from lameness and clinical dysfunction.
- DJD—radiographic evidence in almost all affected stifle joints

MISCELLANEOUS

ASSOCIATED CONDITIONS
Cranial cruciate ligament disease

AGE-RELATED FACTORS
N/A

ZOONOTIC POTENTIAL
N/A

PREGNANCY
N/A

SEE ALSO
Arthritis (Osteoarthritis)

ABBREVIATIONS
DJD = degenerative joint disease
NSAIDs = nonsteroidal antiinflammatory drugs

Suggested Reading
Arnoczky S, Tarvin G. Surgical repair of patella luxations and fractures. In: Bojrab MJ, ed. Current techniques in small animal surgery. 4th ed. Philadelphia: Lea & Febiger, 1998: 1237–1244.

Brinker WO, Piermattei DL, Flo GL. Patellar luxations. In: Brinker WO, Piermattei DL, Flo GL, eds. Handbook of small animal orthopedics and fracture repair. 3rd ed. Philadelphia, Saunders, 1997:516–534.

Slocum B, Slocum TD. Patella luxation. In: Bojrab MJ, ed. Current techniques in small animal surgery. 4th ed. Philadelphia: Lea & Febiger, 1998:1222–1236.

Willauer C, Vasseur P. Clinical results of surgical correction of medial luxation of the patella in dogs. Vet Surg 1987; 16:31–36.

Author: Peter D. Schwarz
Consulting Editor: Peter K. Shires

Polyarthritis, Erosive, Immune-Mediated

 BASICS

DEFINITION
An immune-mediated inflammatory disease of joints that results in erosion of articular cartilage

PATHOPHYSIOLOGY
- Pathogenesis—inciting cause unknown as extrapolated from human rheumatoid arthritis research; likely perpetuated by cell-mediated immunity; predominance of CD4+ helper T lymphocytes and immune complex depositions found in synovium of affected joints; leukocytes, leukocyte enzymes, cell-mediated immunity, immune complexes, and autoallergic reactions are directed against cartilage components; leads to an inflammatory response and complement activation
- Destructive enzymes—released from inflammatory cells, synoviocytes, and chondrocytes; damage the articular cartilage, leading to erosive changes
- IEP—associated with an abnormal antigenic response to host immunoglobulin, similar to human rheumatoid arthritis
- EPG and FCPP—offending antigens unknown

SYSTEMS AFFECTED
Musculoskeletal—diarthrodial joints

GENETICS
Not known to be hereditary

INCIDENCE/PREVALENCE
Rare

GEOGRAPHIC DISTRIBUTION
N/A

POLYARTHRITIS, EROSIVE, IMMUNE-MEDIATED

SIGNALMENT

Species
- Dogs—IEP; EPG
- Cats—FCPP

Breed Predilections
- Small or toy breeds (dogs)—more susceptible to IEP
- Greyhounds—only breed known to be susceptible to EPG

Mean Age and Range
- IEP (dogs)—young to middle-aged (8 months to 8 years)
- EPG—young greyhounds (3–30 months) more susceptible
- FCPP (cats)—onset at 1.5–4.5 years of age

Predominant Sex
FCPP—reported to affect only male cats

SIGNS

General Comments
Nonerosive and erosive forms of immune-mediated inflammatory disease initially appear similar

Historical Findings
- Dogs and cats—initial symmetric stiffness, especially after rest, or intermittent shifting leg lameness and swelling of affected joints
- Cats—may note a more insidious onset; may note shifting leg lameness
- Joint swelling—may be evident, especially in the carpi and tarsi
- Usually no history of trauma
- May also note vomiting, diarrhea, anorexia, pyrexia, depression, and lymphadenopathy
- Often cyclic—may appear to respond to antibiotic therapy, but may be undergoing spontaneous remission

Physical Examination Findings
- Stiffness of gait, lameness, decreased range of motion, crepitus, and joint swelling and pain in one or more joints
- Joint instability, subluxation, and luxation—depend on duration of disease

POLYARTHRITIS, EROSIVE, IMMUNE-MEDIATED

- Lameness—mild weight-bearing to more severe non–weight-bearing
- Diarthrodial joints—all may be affected; IEP and FCPP usually affect the carpi, tarsi, and phalangeal joints; EPG usually affects the carpi, proximal interphalangeal joints, tarsi, elbow, stifle, and hip.

CAUSES
- Unknown
- Immunologic mechanism likely
- *Mycoplasma spumans* (EPG)—cultured from one affected greyhound; not isolated in other patients
- FeLV and FeSFV—linked to cats with FCPP

RISK FACTORS
N/A

 DIAGNOSIS

DIFFERENTIAL DIAGNOSIS
- Idiopathic polyarthritis
- Infectious arthritis
- Systemic lupus erythematosus
- Reactive polyarthritis
- Neoplasia
- Osteoarthritis—primary or secondary

CBC/BIOCHEMISTRY/URINALYSIS
- Usually normal
- Hemogram—may note leukocytosis, neutrophilia, and hyperfibrinogenemia

OTHER LABORATORY TESTS
- Rheumatoid factor—positive in only about 25% of IEP patients
- Coombs' test and antinuclear antibody titer—normal
- Serum titers for *Borrelia*, *Ehrlichia*, and *Rickettsia*—should be normal
- Serologic evidence of FeSFV—found in all FCPP patients
- Serologic evidence of FeLV exposure—found in 50% or fewer of FCPP patients

POLYARTHRITIS, EROSIVE, IMMUNE-MEDIATED

IMAGING

Radiography

- Earliest finding is periarticular soft tissue swelling
- Severe disease—joint capsular distention; osteophytosis; soft tissue thickening; narrowed joint spaces; subchondral sclerosis; decreased trabecular bone density; bony ankylosis in severely affected joints
- Cyst-like lucencies—occasionally seen in subchondral bone
- Chronic disease—subluxation, luxation, and obvious joint deformity

DIAGNOSTIC PROCEDURES

- Arthrocentesis and synovial fluid analysis—essential for diagnosis
- Synovial fluid—typically cloudy with normal viscosity; large number of nondegenerate neutrophils (10,000–100,000 cells/mL); submit for bacterial culture and sensitivity
- Biopsy of synovial tissue—helps make the diagnosis, rules out other arthritides and neoplasia

PATHOLOGIC FINDINGS

- Erosion of articular cartilage—particularly near the periphery at synovial attachments
- Eburnation and sclerosis of subchondral bone with full-thickness cartilage loss—chronic disease
- Synovial membrane—grossly thickened; may see villous projections
- Granulation tissue (pannus)—may invade the margins of articular cartilage, and arise from the marrow cavity to destroy cartilage at central regions of the joint
- Enthesiophytes—at joint capsular attachments and adjacent to the joint
- Histopathology of the synovial membrane—typically reveals villous synovial hyperplasia, hypertrophy, and lymphoplasmacytic inflammatory infiltrate
- Synovial fluid—cloudy; increased volume

TREATMENT

APPROPRIATE HEALTH CARE
Usually outpatient

NURSING CARE
- Physical therapy—range-of-motion exercises, massage, and swimming; may be indicated for severe disease
- Bandages and/or splints—to prevent further breakdown of the joint; may be indicated for severe disease with greatly compromised ambulation

ACTIVITY
Limited to minimize aggravation of clinical signs

DIET
Weight reduction—to decrease stress placed on affected joints

CLIENT EDUCATION
Warn clients of the poor prognosis for cure and complete resolution.

SURGICAL CONSIDERATIONS
- Healing rates—may be long and protracted; range of recovery levels
- Surgery—generally not recommended as a good treatment option
- Arthroplasty—total hip replacement, femoral head ostectomy; may consider
- Arthrodesis—in selective cases of joint pain and joint instability; carpus; generally yields the best results and is a good salvage option; shoulder, elbow, stifle or hock: less predictable results

 ## MEDICATIONS

DRUG(S) OF CHOICE

IEP
- NSAIDs (dogs)—unrewarding
- Prednisone—1.5–2.0 mg/kg PO q12h for 10–14 days as initial therapy; slowly taper over several weeks to 1.0

mg/kg PO q48h if synovial fluid cell counts return to
< 4000 cells/mL and mononuclear cells predominate;
add cytotoxic drugs if clinical signs persist or synovial
fluid analysis is abnormal

- Combination of glucocorticoids and cytotoxic drugs—
  recommended for synergistic effect; may try cyclophosphamide, azathioprine, 6-mercaptopurine, methotrexate,
  or leflunomide
- Cyclophosphamide—patient < 10 kg: 2.5 mg/kg; patient
  10–50 kg: 2.0 mg/kg; patient > 50 kg: 1.75 mg/kg;
  agent given orally q24h for 4 consecutive days of each
  week; can give concurrently with prednisone, the dose of
  prednisone may be decreased by half.
- Azathioprine or 6-mercaptopurine—2.0 mg/kg PO q24h
  for 14–21 days, then give q48h; give prednisone as for
  cyclophosphamide, but on alternating days
- Leflunomide—dog dose 4 mg/kg PO q24h; dosage may
  be adjusted after several days to maintain trough level of
  20 μg/mL.
- Remission—usually induced by combination chemotherapy within 2–16 weeks; determined by resolution of clinical signs and confirmation of a normal synovial fluid
  analysis
- Discontinue cytotoxic drugs 1–3 months after remission
  is achieved.
- Maintaining remission—alternate-day glucocorticoid therapy (prednisone 1.0 mg/kg PO) is generally successful; if
  clinical signs or synovial effusion recurs, may require
  long-term cytotoxic drug therapy; if clinical signs do not
  recur in 2–3 months, may stop the glucocorticoid; if
  clinical signs recur after glucocorticoid is stopped,
  reinstitute treatment
- Aurothiomalate (chrysotherapy)—1 mg/kg IM weekly;
  successfully alleviates symptoms

EPG

- Treatment is unrewarding.
- Antibiotics, NSAIDs, glucocorticoids, cytotoxic drugs, and
  polysulfated glycosaminoglycan (Adequan)—fail to
  induce remission

POLYARTHRITIS, EROSIVE, IMMUNE-MEDIATED

FCPP
- Treatment may help slow progression.
- Prednisone (2 mg/kg q12h) and cyclophosphamide (2.5 mg/kg q24h)—typically used as described for IEP

CONTRAINDICATIONS
- Cytotoxic drugs—do not use with chronic infections or bone marrow suppression (cats with FCPP)
- Chrysotherapy—do not use with renal disease owing to nephrotoxicity

PRECAUTIONS
- Glucocorticoids—long-term use may lead to Cushing's disease
- Cytotoxic drugs—frequently induce bone marrow suppression; monitor CBC: if leukocyte count < 6000 cells/mL and platelet count < 125,000 cells/mL, discontinue for 1 week, then reinstitute at three-quarters dose when counts return to normal
- Thiopurines generally cause bone marrow suppression at 2–6 weeks; cyclophosphamide, at several months.
- Cyclophosphamide—limit to < 4 months; sterile hemorrhagic cystitis may develop; immediately discontinue if symptoms occur
- Leflunomide requires a plasma trough level for monitoring; is intestinally necrotizing to dogs at higher dosages.

POSSIBLE INTERACTIONS
None known

ALTERNATIVE DRUG(S)
See Drugs of Choice

 FOLLOW-UP

PATIENT MONITORING
- Treatment is often frustrating and requires frequent reevaluation.
- Clinical deterioration—requires a change in drug selection or dosage, or surgical intervention

- Important to try to induce remission; allowing the disease to smolder uncontrolled will increase risk of secondary degenerative joint disease

PREVENTION/AVOIDANCE
N/A

POSSIBLE COMPLICATIONS
N/A

EXPECTED COURSE AND PROGNOSIS
- Progression likely
- Long-term prognosis poor
- Cure is not expected; remission is the goal.

 MISCELLANEOUS

ASSOCIATED CONDITIONS
N/A

AGE-RELATED FACTORS
N/A

ZOONOTIC POTENTIAL
N/A

PREGNANCY
N/A

SEE ALSO
Polyarthritis, Nonerosive, Immune-Mediated

ABBREVIATIONS
- EPG = erosive polyarthritis of greyhounds
- FCPP = feline chronic progressive polyarthritis
- FeLV = feline leukemia virus
- FeSFV = feline syncytium-forming virus
- IEP = idiopathic erosive polyarthritis

Suggested Reading
Beale BS. Arthropathies. In: Bloomberg MS, Taylor RT, Dee J, eds. Canine sports medicine and surgery. Philadelphia: Saunders, 1998:517–532.

POLYARTHRITIS, EROSIVE, IMMUNE-MEDIATED

Goring RL, Beale BS. Immune mediated arthritides. In: Bojrab MJ, ed. Disease mechanisms in small animal surgery. Philadelphia: Lea & Febiger, 1993:742–750.

Pedersen NC, Morgan JP, Vasseur PB. Joint diseases of dogs and cats. In: Ettinger SJ, Feldman EC, eds. Textbook of veterinary internal medicine—diseases of the dog and cat. 5th ed. Philadelphia: Saunders, 2000:1862–1886.

Ralphs SC, Beale BS, Whitney WO, Liska W. Idiopathic erosive polyarthritis in six dogs (description of the disease and treatment with bilateral pancarpal arthrodesis). J Vet Comp Orthop Traumatol 2000; 13:191–196.

Ralphs SC, Beale BS. Canine idiopathic erosive polyarthritis. Compendium 2000; 22:671–677, 703.

Authors: Brian Beale and Deanna Worley
Consulting Editor: Peter Shires

Polyarthritis, Nonerosive, Immune-Mediated

 BASICS

DEFINITION
An immune-mediated inflammatory disease of joints that does not cause erosive change; includes idiopathic polyarthritis, SLE, polyarthritis associated with chronic disease (chronic infectious, neoplastic, or enteropathic disease), polyarthritis-polymyositis syndrome, polymyositis syndrome, polyarthritis-meningitis syndrome, polyarthritis nodosa, familial renal amyloidosis in Chinese shar-pei dogs, lymphocytic-plasmacytic synovitis, juvenile-onset polyarthritis of Akitas, and the proliferative form of FCPP

PATHOPHYSIOLOGY
- Pathogenesis—involves a type III hypersensitivity reaction; immune complexes deposited within the synovial membrane; inflammatory response and complement activation ensue, leading to clinical signs of arthritis
- SLE—nuclear material from various cells becomes antigenic, leading to formation of autoantibodies (antinuclear antibody)

SYSTEMS AFFECTED
Musculoskeletal—diarthrodial joints

GENETICS
Not known to be hereditary

INCIDENCE/PREVALENCE
- Idiopathic—most common in dogs
- Other forms uncommon

GEOGRAPHIC DISTRIBUTION
N/A

SIGNALMENT

Species
Dogs and cats

POLYARTHRITIS, NONEROSIVE, IMMUNE-MEDIATED

Breed Predilections
- Idiopathic—large- (more common) and small-breed dogs; uncommon in cats; German shepherds, Doberman pinschers, retrievers, spaniels, pointers, toy poodles, Lhasa apsos, Yorkshire terriers, and Chihuahuas overrepresented
- SLE—tendency to affect large-breed dogs; collies, German shepherds, poodles, terriers, beagles, and Shetland sheepdogs
- Secondary to administration of sulfa drugs—increased sensitivity in Doberman pinschers
- Polyarthritis-meningitis syndrome—reported in weimaraners, German shorthaired pointers, boxers, Bernese mountain dogs, beagles, rottweilers, and Japanese Akitas
- Amyloidosis and synovitis—prominent features of a syndrome affecting young shar-pei dogs
- Juvenile onset—polyarthritis reported in Akitas
- Lymphocytic-plasmacytic synovitis in German shepherds and other large breed dogs

Mean Age and Range
Dogs—young to middle-aged

Predominant Sex
FCPP—male cats only

SIGNS

General Comments
Nonerosive and erosive forms of immune-mediated inflammatory disease initially appear similar

Historical Findings
- Dogs and cats—acute onset; single- or multiple-limb lameness
- Lameness—may shift from leg to leg
- Usually no history of trauma
- May also note vomiting, diarrhea, anorexia, pyrexia, polyuria, or polydypsia
- May also note signs associated with systemic disease or infections (pyometra, prostatitis, or diskospondylitis), or neoplastic disease

- Often cyclic—may appear to respond to antibiotic therapy, but may be undergoing spontaneous remission
- Disease may develop when patient is being treated with (sulfur-containing) antibiotics.

Physical Examination Findings

- Stiffness of gait, lameness, decreased range of motion, crepitus, and joint swelling and pain in one or more joints
- Lameness—mild weight-bearing to more severe non–weight-bearing
- Diarthrodial joints—all may be affected; usually stifle, elbow, carpus, and tarsus

CAUSES

- Unknown for most
- Immunologic mechanism likely
- Chronic—associated with antigenic stimulation along with concurrent meningitis, gastrointestinal disease, neoplasia, urinary tract infection, periodontitis, bacterial endocarditis, heartworm disease, pyometra, chronic otitis media or externa, fungal infections, and chronic *Actinomyces* or *Salmonella* infections
- May occur secondary to a hypersensitivity reaction involving the deposition of drug-antibody complexes in the blood vessels of the synovium; suspected antibiotics include sulfas, cephalosporins, lincomycin, erythromycin, and penicillins.
- FeLV and FeSFV—linked to FCPP

RISK FACTORS

N/A

 DIAGNOSIS

DIFFERENTIAL DIAGNOSIS

- Early erosive polyarthritides
- Infectious arthritis
- Joint trauma
- Polymyositis

POLYARTHRITIS, NONEROSIVE, IMMUNE-MEDIATED

CBC/BIOCHEMISTRY/URINALYSIS
- Usually normal
- Hemogram—may show leukocytosis, neutrophilia, and hyperfibrinogenemia
- Hematologic abnormalities (e.g., thrombocytopenia and hemolytic anemia)—seen in only 10%–20% of patients with SLE

OTHER LABORATORY TESTS
- Positive lupus erythematosus preparation or positive antinuclear antibody test—dogs with SLE
- Serum titers (*Borrelia*, *Ehrlichia*, and *Rickettsia*)—should be normal
- Serologic evidence of FeSFV—found in all FCPP patients
- Serologic evidence of FeLV exposure—found in 50% or fewer of cats with FCPP

IMAGING
- Primary radiographic change—joint capsular distention
- May see enthesiophytosis in prolonged or recurrent disease

DIAGNOSTIC PROCEDURES
- Arthrocentesis and synovial fluid analysis—essential for diagnosis
- Synovial fluid—typically appears cloudy with normal viscosity; large increase in nondegenerate neutrophils (20,000–200,000 cells/mL); submit for bacterial culture and sensitivity
- Synovial biopsy—may help diagnosis

PATHOLOGIC FINDINGS
- Joint capsule—may be thickened; synovial effusion
- Synovial hypertrophy and hyperplasia—associated with a mononuclear cell infiltrate
- Neutrophils—seen in the synovial tissues owing to chemotaxis

 TREATMENT

APPROPRIATE HEALTH CARE
Usually outpatient

NURSING CARE
- Physical therapy—range-of-motion exercises and swimming; may be indicated for severe disease
- Bandages and/or splints—to prevent further breakdown of the joint; may be indicated for severe disease with compromised ambulation

ACTIVITY
Limited to minimize aggravation of clinical signs

DIET
Weight reduction—to decrease stress placed on affected joints

CLIENT EDUCATION
Warn client of poor prognosis for cure and complete resolution.

SURGICAL CONSIDERATIONS
N/A

 MEDICATIONS

DRUG(S) OF CHOICE
- Typical therapy—initial trial of glucocorticoids; if poor response, then combination chemotherapy (glucocorticoids and cytotoxic drugs)
- Eliminate underlying causes if possible—chronic disease; offending antibiotic.
- Complete remission—usually achieved in 2–16 weeks; determined by resolution of clinical signs and confirmation of normal synovial fluid analysis
- Recurrence rate—30%–50% once therapy is discontinued
- Prednisone—1.5–2.0 mg/kg PO q12h for 10–14 days as initial treatment; synovial fluid cell counts < 4000 cells/mL and mononuclear cells predominate: slowly taper over several weeks to 1.0 mg/kg PO q48h; clinical signs persist or abnormal synovial fluid analysis: add cytotoxic agents; no clinical signs after 2–3 months of alternate-day therapy: discontinue

POLYARTHRITIS, NONEROSIVE, IMMUNE-MEDIATED

- Combination of glucocorticoids and cytotoxic drug—recommend for synergistic effect; may try cyclophosphamide or a thiopurine (azathioprine or 6-mercaptopurine)
- Cyclophosphamide—patient < 10 kg: 2.5 mg/kg; patient 10–50 kg: 2.0 mg/kg; patient > 50 kg: 1.75 mg/kg; agent given PO q24h for 4 consecutive days of each week; given concurrently with prednisone (as described above; some clinicians reduce the total steroid dose by half)
- Azathioprine or 6-mercaptopurine—2.0 mg/kg PO q24h for 14–21 days, then q48h; given concurrently with prednisone as for cyclophosphamide, but on alternating days
- Leflunomide—may be used synergistically with azathioprine, prednisone, and cyclophosphamide (4.0 mg/kg q24h for dogs). After several days, adjust dose to plasma trough levels of 20 μg/mL
- Discontinue cytotoxic drugs 1–3 months after remission is achieved.
- Maintaining remission—alternate-day glucocorticoid therapy (prednisone, 1.0 mg/kg PO) is generally successful; clinical signs or synovial neutrophilia recur: long-term cytotoxic drug therapy may be necessary; clinical signs do not recur after 2–3 months: may stop the glucocorticoid; clinical signs recur after glucocorticoid is stopped: continue treatment

FCPP
- Treatment may slow progression
- Prednisone (2 mg/kg q12h) and cyclophosphamide (2.5 mg/kg)—typically as described above

CONTRAINDICATIONS
- Do not use cytotoxic drugs with chronic infections or bone marrow suppression (cats with FCPP)
- Avoid using glucocorticoids with NSAIDs such as aspirin, carprofen, etodolac, and deracoxib as gastric ulceration may result

PRECAUTIONS
- Glucocorticoids—long-term use may lead to iatrogenic Cushing's disease

- Cytotoxic drugs—frequently induce bone marrow suppression; monitor CBC weekly (see Polyarthritis, Erosive, Immune-Mediated)
- Leflunomide may cause intestinal necrosis with overdosing.

POSSIBLE INTERACTIONS
None known

ALTERNATIVE DRUG(S)
See Drugs of Choice.

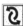 **FOLLOW-UP**

PATIENT MONITORING
Clinical deterioration—indicates a change in drug selection or dosage

PREVENTION/AVOIDANCE
N/A

POSSIBLE COMPLICATIONS
N/A

EXPECTED COURSE AND PROGNOSIS
- Recurrence—seen intermittently
- SLE and FCPP—progression common; guarded prognosis
- Other forms—good prognosis

 MISCELLANEOUS

ASSOCIATED CONDITIONS
N/A

AGE-RELATED FACTORS
N/A

ZOONOTIC POTENTIAL
N/A

PREGNANCY
N/A

POLYARTHRITIS, NONEROSIVE, IMMUNE-MEDIATED

ABBREVIATIONS

- FCPP = feline chronic progressive polyarthritis
- FeLV = feline leukemia virus
- FeSFV = feline syncytium-forming virus
- SLE = systemic lupus erythematosus
- NSAID = nonsteroidal antiinflammatory drug

Suggested Reading

Beale BS. Arthropathies. In: Bloomberg MS, Taylor RT, Dee J, eds. Canine sports medicine and surgery. Philadelphia: Saunders, 1998:517–532.

Goring RL, Beale BS. Immune mediated arthritides. In: Bojrab MJ, ed. Disease mechanisms in small animal surgery. Philadelphia: Lea & Febiger, 1993:742–750.

Pedersen NC. Joint diseases of dogs and cats. In: Ettinger SJ, ed. Textbook of veterinary internal medicine. 5th ed. Philadelphia: Saunders, 2000:1862–1886.

Authors: Brian S. Beale and Scott P. Hammel
Consulting Editor: Peter Shires

Shoulder, Ligament, and Tendon Conditions

 BASICS

DEFINITION
- Make up the majority of causes for lameness in the canine shoulder joint, excluding osteochondritis dissecans lesions

PATHOPHYSIOLOGY

Bicipital Tenosynovitis
- Strain injury to the tendon of the biceps brachii
- Mechanism of injury—direct trauma; indirect trauma (more common)
- Pathologic changes—from partial disruption of the tendon to chronic inflammatory changes, including dystrophic calcification
- Proliferation of the fibrous connective tissue and adhesions between the tendon and the sheath—limit motion; cause pain

Fibrotic Contracture of the Infraspinatus Muscle
- Primary muscle–tendon disorder—not a neuropathy
- Fibrous tissue—replaces normal muscle–tendon unit architecture
- Loss of elasticity
- Functional shortening of the muscle and tendon
- Degeneration and atrophy of affected muscle
- Partial muscle disruption—likely caused by direct or indirect trauma

Other
- Rupture of the biceps brachii tendon of origin—strain injury or disruption of the tendinous fibers at or near the junction with the supraglenoid tubercle of the scapula
- Mineralization of the supraspinatus tendon— degenerative condition; granular grayish white calcium deposited between the fibers of the tendon; unknown cause; probably the result of overuse and indirect trauma

SHOULDER, LIGAMENT, AND TENDON CONDITIONS

- Avulsion or fracture of the supraspinatus tendon—overuse injury; variable amount of bone is avulsed from the greater tubercle of the proximal humerus

SYSTEMS AFFECTED
Musculoskeletal

INCIDENCE/PREVALENCE
Common cause of forelimb lameness

SIGNALMENT

Species
Dogs

Breed Predilections
Medium- to large-breed dogs

Mean Age and Range
- Skeletally mature dogs ≥ 1 year of age
- Usually 3–7 years of age

SIGNS

General Comments
- Depend on the severity and chronicity of the disease
- Atrophy of the spinati muscles—consistent finding for all conditions

Historical Findings
- Bicipital tenosynovitis—onset usually insidious; often of several months' duration; may be a traumatic incident as the inciting cause; subtle, intermittent lameness that worsens with exercise
- Rupture of the biceps brachii tendon of origin—similar to bicipital tenosynovitis; may have acute onset due to a known traumatic event; usually subtle, chronic lameness that worsens with exercise
- Mineralization of the supraspinatus tendon—onset usually insidious; chronic lameness that worsens with activity
- Avulsion/fracture of the supraspinatus tendon—similar to mineralization of supraspinatus tendon

SHOULDER, LIGAMENT, AND TENDON CONDITIONS

- Fibrotic contracture of the infraspinatus muscle—usually sudden onset during a period of outdoor exercise (e.g., hunting); shoulder lameness and tenderness gradually disappears within 2 weeks; condition results in chronic, persistent lameness 3–4 weeks later, which is not particularly painful

Physical Examination Findings
- Bicipital tenosynovitis—short and limited swing phase of gait owing to pain on extension and flexion of the shoulder; pain inconsistently demonstrated on manipulation of shoulder; pain most evident by applying deep digital pressure over the tendon in the intertubercular groove region while simultaneously flexing the shoulder and extending the elbow
- Rupture of the biceps brachii tendon—similar
- Mineralization of the supraspinatus tendon—similar; manipulations often do not produce pain; may palpate firm swelling over the greater tubercle
- Avulsion or fracture of the supraspinatus tendon—similar to mineralization of the supraspinatus tendon
- Fibrotic contracture of the infraspinatus muscle—usually not painful on manipulation; internal rotation (pronation) of the shoulder joint—patient incapable; when forced, caudal aspect of the scapula elevates off the trunk and becomes more prominent, when patient is standing—elbow adducted; paw abducted and outwardly rotated; when patient is walking—lower limb swings in a lateral arc (circumduction) as the paw is advanced during the stride; marked atrophy of the infraspinatus muscle on palpation

CAUSES
- Indirect or direct trauma—likely
- Strain injury (indirect trauma)—most common

RISK FACTORS
- Overexertion
- Poor conditioning before performing athletic activities
- Obesity

SHOULDER, LIGAMENT, AND TENDON CONDITIONS

 DIAGNOSIS

DIFFERENTIAL DIAGNOSIS
- Luxation or subluxation of the shoulder joint—often a history of trauma with an acute onset of lameness; often severe lameness with marked pain on manipulation of the shoulder joint
- Osteosarcoma of the proximal humerus—progressive lameness with varying degrees of pain on manipulation of the shoulder; may note swelling and tenderness of the proximal humerus
- Brachial plexus nerve sheath tumor—slow, insidious, progressive lameness over a period of months; marked atrophy of the spinati muscles with chronic disease; may feel a firm mass deep in the axillary region that is painful to digital pressure

IMAGING

Radiology
- Required for differentiation
- Craniocaudal and mediolateral views necessary for all patients

Bicipital Tenosynovitis
- Generally normal
- Mediolateral view (chronic disease)—reveals bony reaction on the supraglenoid tubercle, dystrophic calcification of the bicipital tendon, sclerosis of the floor of the intertubercular groove, and osteophytes in the intertubercular groove
- Hyperflexed CP-CD or CD-CP view (tangential) of the intertubercular groove—important for identifying the location of calcification; CP-CD view taken with patient in sternal recumbency (radiographic cassette placed on top of the forearm) with the elbow hyperflexed; CD-CP view taken with patient in dorsal recumbency with the shoulder joint hyperflexed and the limb rotated externally approximately 30°; position the radiographic tube directly over the scapulohumeral joint

SHOULDER, LIGAMENT, AND TENDON CONDITIONS

Rupture of the Biceps Brachii Tendon of Origin
- Normal
- Chronic disease—may see bony, irregular reaction on the supraglenoid tubercle

Mineralization of the Supraspinatus Tendon
- Mediolateral view—generally reveals calcification
- Occurs cranial and immediately medial to the greater tubercle of the proximal humerus
- Superimposition on the greater tubercle of the humerus—requires high-quality images
- Tangential or skyline view of the intertubercular region of the proximal humerus—as for bicipital tenosynovitis; eliminates superimposition; allows distinction from calcification of the biceps brachii tendon
- Density(ies)—smooth or irregular; multiple lesions common
- Often bilateral radiographically but rarely produces bilateral lameness

Avulsion/Fracture of the Supraspinatus Tendon
- Similar to mineralization of the supraspinatus tendon
- Bone fragment—origin may be seen as a defect in the greater tubercle of the humerus; generally not as radiographically dense as that identified with mineralization of the supraspinatus tendon

Fibrotic Contracture of the Infraspinatus Muscle
Radiographically normal

Ultrasonography
- May help identify bicipital tenosynovitis and rupture of the biceps brachii tendon of origin

Contrast Arthrography
- Helps identify bicipital tenosynovitis
- Useful for determining the location of calcific densities near the intertubercular groove
- Incomplete filling of the tendon sheath—may indicate proliferative inflammatory synovitis and adhesions between the tendon sheath and intertubercular groove

SHOULDER, LIGAMENT, AND TENDON CONDITIONS

DIAGNOSTIC PROCEDURES
- Joint tap and analysis of synovial fluid—identify intraarticular disease; fluid should be straw colored with normal to decreased viscosity; cytologic evaluation: < 10,000 nucleated cells/ml (> 90% are mononuclear cells)
- Arthroscopic exploration of the shoulder joint—diagnose bicipital tenosynovitis and rupture of the biceps brachii tendon of origin; confirm lack of intraarticular disease

PATHOLOGIC FINDINGS
- Bicipital tenosynovitis—grossly, mineralization of the biceps tendon; osteophytosis of the intertubercular groove; proliferative synovitis; and fibrous adhesions between the biceps tendon and its synovial sheath; histologically, synovial proliferation, edema, fibrosis, dystrophic mineralization, and lymphocytic-plasmacytic infiltration of the tendon and synovium
- Rupture of the biceps brachii tendon of origin—grossly, partial to complete rupture of the biceps tendon at its insertion on the supraglenoid tubercle, proliferative synovitis, and fibrous adhesions between the biceps tendon and its synovial sheath; histologically, synovial proliferation, edema, fibrosis, and occasional dystrophic mineralization
- Mineralization of the supraspinatus tendon—grossly, tendon often looks normal, but longitudinal incision reveals numerous pockets of mineralized debris within the fibers; histologically, chondromucinous stromal degeneration of the tendon with multiple foci of dystrophic mineralization
- Avulsion or fracture of the supraspinatus tendon—grossly, tendon often looks normal, but longitudinal incision reveals bone fragment(s) surrounded by a fibrous tissue capsule; usually see a corresponding bony defect in the greater tubercle
- Fibrotic contracture of the infraspinatus muscle—grossly, atrophied, fibrotic, and contracted muscle, normal tendon, and (commonly) adhesions to the underlying joint capsule; histologically, degeneration, atrophy, and fibroplasia within the damaged muscle

TREATMENT

APPROPRIATE HEALTH CARE
- Outpatient—early diagnosis
- Inpatient—chronic, severe disease requires surgical intervention.
- Bicipital tenosynovitis—50%–75% success with medical treatment; requires surgery with evidence of chronic changes and failure of medical management
- Rupture of the biceps brachii tendon of origin generally requires surgery
- Mineralization of the supraspinatus tendon—may be an incidental finding; requires surgery after excluding other causes of lameness and medical treatment
- Avulsion or fracture of the supraspinatus tendon—often requires surgery because of persistent bone fragment irritation of the tendon
- Fibrotic contracture of the infraspinatus muscle—requires surgery

NURSING CARE
- Cryotherapy (ice packing)—immediately postsurgery; helps reduce inflammation and swelling at the surgery site; performed 15–20 min every 8 hr for 3–5 days
- Regional massage and range-of-motion exercises—improve flexibility; decrease muscle atrophy

ACTIVITY
- Medical treatment—requires strict confinement for 4–6 weeks; activity; premature return to normal likely exacerbates signs and induces a chronic state.
- Postsurgery— depends on procedure performed

DIET
Weight control—decrease the load applied to the painful joint

SURGICAL CONSIDERATIONS
- Bicipital tenosynovitis—recommended with poor response to medical treatment and chronic disease; goal: eliminate movement of the biceps tendon within the inflamed synovial sheath by performing a tenodesis of

the bicipital tendon; remove the tendon from its origin on the scapular supraglenoid tubercle and reattach it to the proximal lateral aspect of the humerus.

- Rupture of the biceps brachii tendon of origin—tenodesis is the treatment of choice; reattach tendon to the proximal lateral aspect of the humerus using either a screw and spiked washer or passing the tendon through a bone tunnel and suturing it to the supraspinatus tendon.
- Mineralization of the supraspinatus tendon—longitudinally incise the tendon; remove the calcium deposits.
- Avulsion or fracture of the supraspinatus tendon— remove the bone fragment(s)
- Fibrotic contracture of the infraspinatus muscle—tenotomy and excision of part of the tendon of insertion; often feel a distinct pop after excision of the last adhesion, which allows complete range of motion of the shoulder joint.

 MEDICATIONS

DRUG(S) OF CHOICE

Bicipital Tenosynovitis
- Intraarticular injection of a corticosteroid—initial treatment of choice
- Systemic treatment (NSAIDs or steroids)—not as effective
- Do not inject into a septic joint; perform complete synovial fluid analysis if any doubt.
- Prednisolone acetate—20–40 mg, depending on size
- Lameness markedly improved but not eliminated—give a second injection in 3–6 weeks
- Incomplete resolution—recommend surgery

NSAIDs and Analgesics
- May be used for symptomatic treatment
- May try buffered or enteric-coated aspirin (10–25 mg/kg PO q8–12h), carprofen (2.2 mg/kg PO q12h), etodolac (10–15 mg/kg PO q24h), phenylbutazone (3–7 mg/kg PO q8h, total dose < 800 mg/day), meclofenamic acid (0.5 mg/kg PO q12h), piroxicam (0.3 mg/kg PO q24h for 3 days, then q48h), or deracoxib (3-4 mg/kg PO q24h for 7

days for postoperative pain) (1–2 mg/kg PO q24h for long-term treatment over 7 days)

CONTRAINDICATIONS
- Avoid corticosteroids because of the potential side effects and articular cartilage damage associated with long-term use.
- Direct injection of a corticosteroid into the biceps tendon—may promote further tendon disruption and eventual rupture

PRECAUTIONS
NSAIDs—gastrointestinal irritation may preclude use.

ALTERNATIVE DRUG(S)
Chondroprotective drugs (e.g., polysulfated glycosaminogly-cans, glucosamine, and chondroitin sulfate)—may help limit associated cartilage damage and degeneration

 FOLLOW-UP

PATIENT MONITORING
- Most patients require a minimum of 1–2 months of rehabilitation after treatment.

EXPECTED COURSE AND PROGNOSIS
- Medically managed bicipital tenosynovitis—often successful after one or two treatments (50%–75% of cases) with no chronic changes
- Surgically treated bicipital tenosynovitis—good to excellent results (90% of cases); recovery to full function may take 2–8 months
- Surgically treated tenodesis of the bicipital brachii tendon—good to excellent prognosis; > 85% of patients show improved return to function.
- Surgically treated mineralization of the supraspinatus tendon—good to excellent prognosis; recurrence possible but uncommon
- Surgically treated avulsion or fracture of the supraspinatus tendon—good to excellent prognosis; recurrence possible but uncommon

SHOULDER, LIGAMENT, AND TENDON CONDITIONS

- Surgically treated fibrotic contracture of the infraspinatus muscle—good to excellent prognosis; patients uniformly return to normal limb function

 MISCELLANEOUS

ABBREVIATIONS
CD = craniodorsal
CP = cranioposterior
NSAID = nonsteroidal antiinflammatory drug

Suggested Reading
Flo GL, Middleton D. Mineralization of the supraspinatus tendons in dogs. J Am Vet Med Assoc 1990:197:95–97.
Rivers B, Wallace L, Johnston GR. Biceps tenosynovitis in the dog: radiographic and sonographic findings. Vet Comp Orthop Trauma 1992;5:51–57.
Stobie D, Wallace LJ, Lipowitz AJ, et al. Chronic bicipital tenosynovitis in dogs: 29 cases (1985–1992). J Am Vet Med Assoc 1995;207:201–207.

Author: Peter D. Schwarz
Consulting Editor: Peter K. Shires

Recommended Parenteral NSAID Dosages and Indications

NSAID	Dosage/Route/Duration	Indications	Comments
Carprofen (injectable)	Dog: 2–4 mg/kg IV, SC q24hr Cat: 1.0 mg/kg SC only once	Mild to moderate pain	Primarily used perioperatively before switching to oral formulation; GI irritation and altered renal function
Meloxicam (injectable)	Dog: 0.2 mg/kg initially IM, IV, or SC; 0.1 mg/kg thereafter SC Cat: 0.1–0.2 mg/kg initially IM, IV, or SC; 0.05–0.1 mg/kg thereafter SC Duration: 24 hr	Mild to moderate pain	Can be mixed with food; GI irritation and altered renal function
Ketoprofen (injectable)	Dog: 1.0–2.0 mg/kg initially IM, IV, or SC; 0.5–1.0 mg/kg thereafter SC Cat: 1.0–2.0 mg/kg initially IM, IV, or SC; 0.5–1.0 mg/kg thereafter SC Duration: 24 hr	Mild to moderate pain; in Canada for dogs and cats and in the U.S. for horses	GI irritation and altered renal function. Dosing should not exceed 5 days for dogs and 3 days for cats

GI = gastrointestinal; NSAID = nonsteroidal anti-inflammatory drug.

Recommended Dispensable NSAID Dosages and Indications

NSAID	Dosage/Route/Duration	Indications	Comments
Carprofen (tablets and chewables)	Dog: 1.0–2.0 mg/kg PO q24hr Cat: 1.0 mg/kg PO (1 dose only) Duration: 12–24 hr	Mild to moderate pain; approved in the U.S. for dogs	Toxicity associated with chronic use in cats; minimal toxicity in dogs with chronic use, but may cause GI irritation and altered renal function in some patients
Deracoxib (chewable tablets)	Dog (postoperative pain): 3.0–4.0 mg/kg q24hr as needed for 7 days Dog (osteoarthritis): 1–2 mg/kg PO q24hr for long-term treatment over 7 days Duration: 24 hr	Pain and inflammation associated with osteoarthritis. Postoperative pain and inflammation associated with orthopedic surgery in dogs with osteoarthritis. Postoperative >1.8 kg; approved in the U.S.	GI irritation and altered renal function

Drug	Dosage	Indications	Comments
Tepoxalin (oral lyophilisate)	Dog: 10–20 mg/kg PO initially; 10 mg/kg thereafter Cat: not used Duration: 24 hr	Mild to moderate pain and inflammation; approved for dogs in the U.S.; perioperative administration not recommended	GI irritation and altered renal function. Dual inhibitor of the 5-LO and COX enzymes; 7-day washout recommended when switching from another NSAID
Etodolac (tablets)	Dog: 10–15 mg/kg PO Cat: not used Duration: 24 hr	Mild to moderate pain; approved for dogs in the U.S.	Hypoproteinemia; GI irritation and altered renal function
Aspirin (tablets)	Dog: 10–25 mg/kg PO Cat: 10–15 mg/kg PO Duration: 6–12 hr for dogs, 24–72 hr for cats	Mild to moderate pain and inflammation	GI irritation and altered renal function; more likely at higher doses
Mefoxicam (oral liquid suspension)	Dog: 0.2 mg/kg initially PO; 0.1 mg/kg thereafter PO Cat: 0.1–0.2 mg/kg initially PO; 0.05–0.1 mg/kg thereafter PO Duration: 24 hr	Mild to moderate pain; approved for dogs in Canada	GI irritation; can be mixed with food. Cats should not be given meloxicam for >5 days.

Recommended Dispensable NSAID Dosages and Indications (cont.)

NSAID	Dosage/Route/Duration	Indications	Comments
Ketoprofen (tablets)	Dog: 1.0–2.0 mg/kg initially PO; 0.5–1.0 mg/kg thereafter PO Cat: 1.0–2.0 mg/kg initially PO; 0.5–1.0 mg/kg thereafter PO Duration: 24 hr	Mild to moderate pain; approved in Canada for dogs and cats and in the U.S. for horses	GI irritation and altered renal functions. Limit administration to 5 days for both dogs and cats
Acetaminophen (tablets and oral liquid suspension)	Dog: 10–15 mg/kg PO Cat: contraindicated Duration (in dogs): 8–12 hr	Mild to moderate pain; low anti-inflammatory action	Toxic to cats; often given in combination with codeine to dogs (see oral analgesic preparations)

GI = gastrointestinal; NSAID = nonsteroidal anti-inflammatory drug.

Index

A

INDEX

M

INDEX